(THE BASIC BOOK)

YOGA

E TAI CHI

(Yogetaichi)

**The World's Simplest Yoga-Tai Chi
for All Ages**

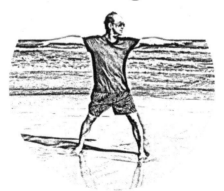

Developed, Written, and Demonstrated by

Yongxin Li, M.D., Ph.D.

Internal Medicine Physician

Copyright

Yoga E Tai Chi
(The Basic Book)

The World's Simplest Yoga-Tai Chi

First Edition: December 2017
(Updated January 2019)

E Tai Chi Logo

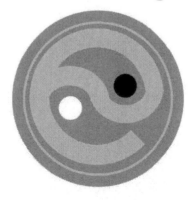

This book is dedicated to:

My wife, Jo, who, my first E Tai Chi student, teaches me yoga;
My children, Jason and Megan, who are my hope;
Dad, Shanquan, who said to me, "You won't achieve anything if
you don't keep fit."

Educational Disclaimer

The medicine and Yoga E Tai Chi described in this book can be viewed as common medical knowledge and a guide to exercises. The movements or postures in Yoga E Tai Chi are scientifically designed and have been applied to my patients safely. Since they involve only gentle hand/arm movements and normal walking or standing, they should not pose a greater risk of injury than people's normal daily activities do. Nevertheless, any exercise can cause potential injuries. You should consult a qualified medical professional before starting a new exercise such as **Yoga E Tai Chi**. The author disclaims any and all liability for damages resulting from the use of information in this book.

Yogetaichi Song

Learning simple yoga-tai chi is so easy,
Walking sideways won't hurt your knee,
Relaxing and stretching reduce pain and stress,
Breathing exercises soothe your mind immensely.

Things are never perfect,
Life is short and hectic.
Let's practice Yogetaichi,
Keep fit and be happy.

By Yongxin Li

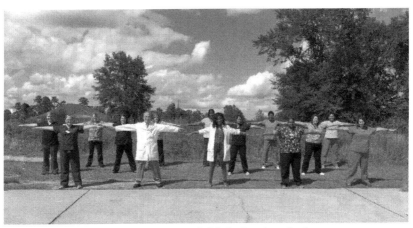

Practicing Yogetaichi during break times.

Pictured from left to right are (first row) Ashley Harris, Yongxin Li, Melanie Sheppard, Charlotte Shuler, and Ann Hawkins; (second row) Kayla Easterlin, Amanda White, Jami Odom, and Sarah Miller; (third row) Amy Coleman, Carolyn Dewitt, Trista Bonnette, Sylvia Rush, and Shadana Carson.

****

Also by Dr. Yongxin Li

Life and Medicine

E Tai Chi (The Basic Book)

E Tai Chi (The Basic Book-Chinese Edition)

E Tai Chi (The Complete Book)

Bicircular E Tai Chi (The Basic Book)

Bicircular E Tai Chi (The Advanced Book)
At Amazon.com

Yoga E Tai Chi (The Advanced Book)

E Tai Chi (The Science Book)
Coming soon.

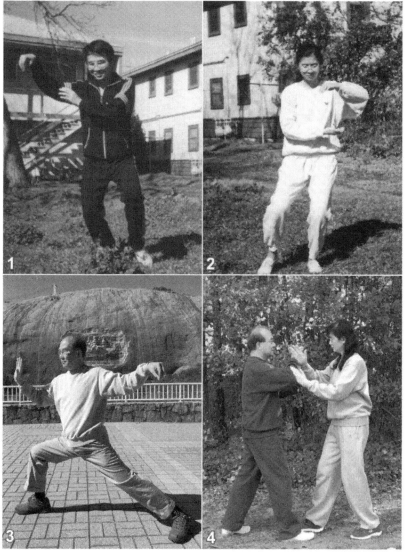

Photos #1 and **#2**: Jo, my wife, and I practiced tai chi in Galveston, Texas, in 1986.

Photos #3 and **#4**: Today, three decades later, tai chi remains one of our favorite exercises.

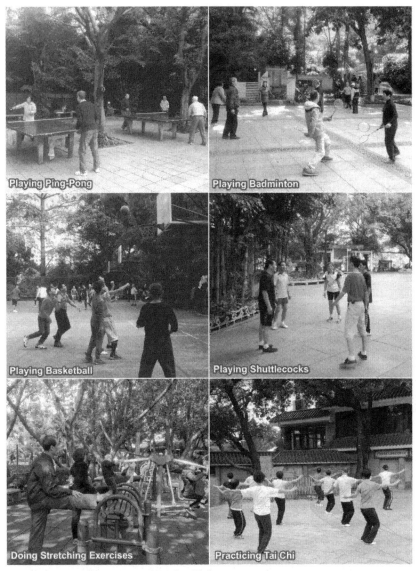

Various outdoor exercises in China.

Practicing tai chi is just one of the many morning exercises Chinese people do in the park.

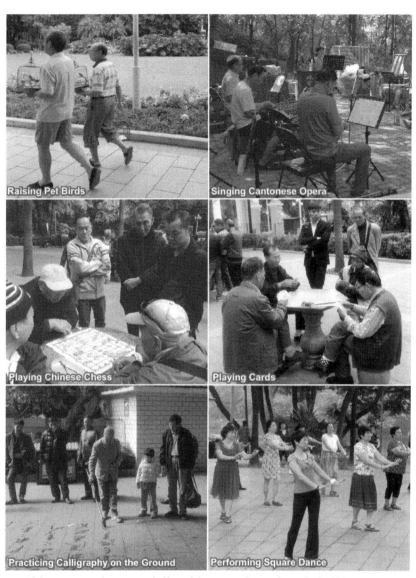

Chinese people, especially older people, enjoy their life through a variety of activities.

List of Videos

(These videos are embedded in the Kindle eBook version of the book.)

The video recordings have been compressed to save space. Thus, the video images in the book may have a lower resolution than the original. All the videos are played back at the original recording speed.

Basic E Tai Chi Sequence (Page 64)

Hand/Arm Moments 1, 2, 3, 4, 5, and **6** (Page 112)

Standing Yoga E Tai Chi Postures
Upward Movement 1 and Forward Movement 1 (Page 129)
Sideward Movements 1, 2, and 3 (Page 139)
Downward Movement 2 and Backward Movement 2 (Page 151)
Balance Movements 1a, 1b, 2, and 3 (Page 163)

Basic Yoga E Tai Chi Walking Sequence (Page 76)
Starting Posture and Posture One (Page 181)
Posture Two and Posture Three (Page 194)
Postures Four/Five and Closing Posture-Front View (Page 205)
Postures Four/Five and Closing Posture-Lateral View (Page 205)

Also, you can watch the videos of E Tai Chi and Yoga E Tai Chi sequences demonstrated by the author on YouTube:
Yoga E Tai Chi (the basic postures and sequence)
https://www.youtube.com//watch?v=iU1ceeKs0JY
E Tai Chi (the basic sequence)
https://www.youtube.com/watch?v=QjbVILwHwCY
E Tai Chi (the intermediate and advanced sequences)
https://www.youtube.com/watch?v=Medo50cBNEc

Table of Contents

Author's Note

大道至简

The greatest truths are the simplest.
—老子 (Lao Tzu, 571 B.C., Chinese philosopher)

Simplicity is the ultimate sophistication.
—Leonardo da Vinci (1452 –1519, Italian Renaissance polymath)

This is a book about a combination exercise of yoga and tai chi. Please read another book of mine, *E Tai Chi (The Basic Book),* if you are interested in genuine tai chi.

Tai chi is also known as **Tai Chi Chuan** or **Taijiquan**, one form of Chinese martial arts, which is characterized by its tranquility, slowness, relaxation, smoothness, and continuity. It is a combination of physical and mental exercises and has been proven to provide many health benefits, e.g., reducing stress, preventing falls, and improving some chronic medical disorders including hypertension, depression, fibromyalgia, and other chronic pain conditions.

E Tai Chi (**Ease** or **Easy Tai Chi**) is a new tai chi fitness system that is scientifically created by the author for the purpose of simplicity, safety, and efficacy. E Tai Chi is the world's simplest and safest tai chi exercise. It consists of sequences of simple and gentle circular hand/arm movements performed with normal walking or standing.

Yoga E Tai Chi is a yoga-tai chi combination exercise that is developed by the author on the basis of E Tai Chi. Namely, you practice yoga by using the E Tai Chi hand/arm movements, stances, and footwork. It does not mean that you perform yoga poses and tai chi postures alternately. Yoga E Tai Chi is E Tai Chi that is practiced in a

yoga-tai chi way. In other words, each of the Yoga E Tai Chi postures is made of both yoga and tai chi components. I name this unique, innovative exercise "**Yogetaichi** (/ˈjoʊgiˈtaɪˈtʃi/ or yoh gee tahy chee)."

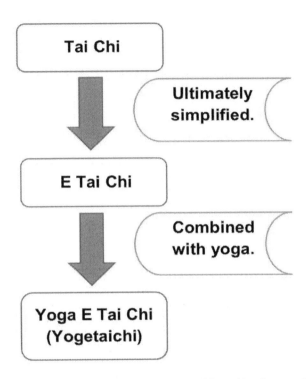

Yoga E Tai Chi is unique, original, scientific, effective, and infinite! It is for personal health only, not for fighting or any spiritual purpose. Its characteristics can be summarized by Five S's: **Simplicity**, **Science**, **Safety**, **Serenity**, and **Strength**.

Simplicity.

The hand/arm movements in yoga and tai chi have been condensed to only **ONE** circular movement, which gives rise to six basic hand/arm movements readily. Therefore, Yoga E Tai Chi is the **ultimate simplest** yoga-tai chi combination exercise that cannot be simplified any more. You do not need yoga uniforms, yoga mats, or other supporting materials. You can practice it anywhere and anytime.

In **Yoga E Tai Chi**, you practice the same hand/arm movements and sequences that are used in E Tai Chi. Of course, some safe and effective yoga components are integrated into those E Tai Chi movements and sequences. If you have mastered E Tai Chi, then you can pick up Yoga E Tai Chi within a couple of hours. You can still learn Yoga E Tai Chi by reading this book and the accompanying videos if you do not know E Tai Chi at all.

Science.

Yoga E Tai Chi is a yoga-tai chi fitness routine that is developed on the basis of E Tai Chi. Specifically, E Tai Chi assimilates the typical elements of yoga: holding poses and stretching fully. Thus, you can find both yoga and tai chi components in each of the Yoga E Tai Chi postures. **Distinctively, you keep rotating your arms/shoulders while you are staying in a pose.** This unique feature that can **only be seen** in Yoga E Tai Chi enhances the efficacy of yoga stretching, maintains the continuity of tai chi postures, and synchronizes your breathing with the hand movements seamlessly.

Not only can you practice Yoga E Tai Chi while standing (performing standing postures), but also while walking (executing walking sequences). Yoga-E Tai Chi maintains the characteristics of tai chi: relaxation, smoothness, and continuity. At the same time, it integrates the unique features of yoga without its shortcomings, such as being difficult to learn, causing injuries easily, etc.

Safety.

The typical tai chi walk, the curved footwork, has been replaced by regular walking or slowed natural walking in E Tai Chi. You do not make turns, squat, or kick. There is no extreme bending, twisting, or upside-down inversion of the body. Because you walk sideways in most of the postures, you can avoid over-flexion of the knees and maintain proper knee/foot alignment.

Only several safe and effective standing yoga poses, which have been modified, are included. Yoga E Tai Chi is especially suitable for older people because a lot of floor or balance poses in common yoga practices are unsafe for them (Swain & McGwin, 2016).

You can practice Yoga E Tai Chi safely anywhere, anytime, during normal walking, and in any position (sitting, standing, or even lying).

Serenity.

Breathing exercises have been proven to be able to soothe one's mind. Even though breathing exercises are emphasized in Yoga E Tai Chi, only **ONE** breathing technique is recommended: conscious natural breathing coordinated with hand/arm movements. It can be mastered and practiced easily because most of the hand/arm movements in Yoga E Tai Chi are symmetrical. You can always follow the simple rule: inhale when raising your hands (or the leading hand) and exhale when lowering your hands (or the leading hand). Similarly, breathe in when turning the palms upward/forward and breathe out when turning the palms downward/backward.

Strength.

In the Yoga E Tai Chi sequences, the majority of the postures involve walking sideways. Yoga E Tai Chi provides an efficient physical workout because sideways walking consumes over three times more energy than forward walking (Handford & Srinivasan, 2014). You can tone up your muscles by holding poses for a more extended period of time or wearing weights on your wrists and ankles. Moreover, you may even turn Yoga E Tai Chi into an aerobic exercise if you practice it at a fast pace.

As is the case with E Tai Chi, you can create your own Yoga E Tai Chi sequences by using the six basic hand movements and different ways of walking or standing. In addition, you can practice Yoga E Tai Chi postures and pure E Tai Chi postures alternately in a sequence. Yoga E Tai Chi relaxes your body, reduces stress, promotes physical fitness, and cultivates the sensation of feeling good. Since Yoga E Tai Chi is simple and safe, you can easily incorporate it into your day to day life. I can guarantee that you will feel refreshed and energized after 5-10 minutes of Yoga E Tai Chi practice. If you want to practice both tai chi and yoga to improve your health, then Yoga E Tai Chi is the only tai chi and yoga exercise you need for the rest of your life.

In this book, I have tried to focus on teaching how to learn Yoga E Tai Chi quickly and to perform it safely as opposed to discussing the mysterious and scientifically unproven theories about traditional tai chi and yoga (e.g., qi, prana, and chakras). People that are interested in those topics can read other tai chi or yoga books. Also, you can learn about my views on Chinese medicine in my book (*Life and Medicine, Chapter 6, Seeing Doctors in China*). All major statements in the book are supported by the attached references or the relevant Wikipedia articles. By using common sense, we know that any moderate, safe, and regular exercise will have health benefits. In the 21st century, what we need is science, peace, prosperity, and health.

This is the only book from which you can learn yoga-tai chi by yourself. It contains more detailed illustrations than any yoga or tai chi books on the market. The arrows that are added to almost all the figures in the book indicate the direction of hand and foot movements. The systematic flowcharts show where you go, how many steps you walk, and how you move your feet. In the course of learning a new posture, you will be given clear instructions on when to inhale and when to exhale.

I use at least nine photos to illustrate each yoga-tai chi movement or posture. I try to provide front views and lateral views of each posture and detailed explanations for the transitions of postures, which are the most difficult to learn. Some of the descriptions, illustrations, and flowcharts are repeated in some sections so that you can have a complete instruction for each movement without reference to other chapters. The e-book version also contains video recordings of all the Yoga E Tai Chi hand/arm movements, postures, and sequences. Additionally, the walking sequences of Yoga E Tai Chi or E Tai Chi demonstrated by the author can be watched on YouTube.

In order to make the learning process simple and not to overwhelm the readers with numerous figures and instructions, I am going to publish two books about Yoga E Tai Chi: the basic book and the advanced book. The advanced book of Yoga E Tai Chi covers the intermediate and advanced Yoga E Tai Chi. Tai chi or yoga beginners can read the basic book first. They can study the advanced book when they become familiar with the basic Yoga E Tai Chi.

As a matter of fact, if you can practice all the exercises described in the basic book daily or 3-4 times per week for 30-40 minutes, then you have already achieved most of the health benefits of yoga and tai chi. Surely, you will appreciate the elegance, ingenuity, and versatility of Yoga E Tai Chi if you read the advanced book.

The first four chapters of my E Tai Chi books covering the basics of E Tai Chi are included in this book. Thus, the readers without knowledge of E Tai Chi can still learn Yoga E Tai Chi by just reading this book. If you have read my E Tai Chi books, then you can start with Chapter 5 after reading **Tai Chi versus Yoga** in Chapter 1, **Yoga E Tai Chi** in Chapter 2, and **Breathing** in Chapter 3.

The Basic Book (242 pages with over 600 photos)
Introduction
Chapter 1. Demystifying Tai Chi
Chapter 2. Characteristics of E Tai Chi and Yoga E Tai Chi
Chapter 3. Basics of E Tai Chi (also used in Yoga E Tai Chi)
Chapter 4. Hand/Arm Movements (1-3)
Chapter 5. Basic Standing Postures in Yoga E Tai Chi
Chapter 6. Basic Walking Sequence in Yoga E Tai Chi

The Advanced Book (> 200 pages):
Introduction (Omitted)
Chapter 1. Demystifying Tai Chi (Omitted)
Chapter 2. Characteristics(Omitted)
Chapter 6. Basic Walking Sequence (Omitted).

Chapter 3. Basics of E Tai Chi (also used in Yoga E Tai Chi)
Chapter 4. Hand/Arm Movements (**1-6**)
Chapter 5. Standing Postures (**more postures**) in Yoga E Tai Chi
Chapter 7. **Intermediate** Walking Sequence in Yoga E Tai Chi
Chapter 8. **Advanced** Yoga E Tai Chi

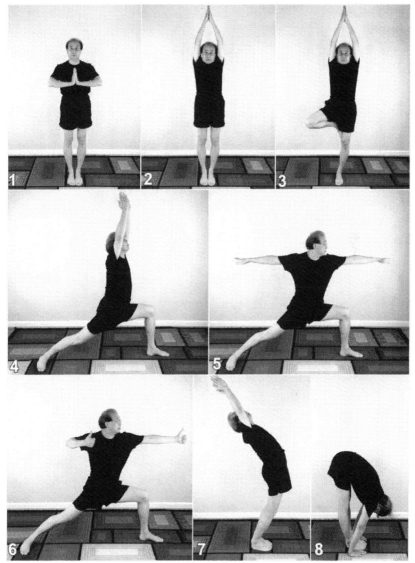

Figure 0-0. Eight yoga poses are adopted in the basic Yoga E Tai Chi.

Photo #1: Mountain Pose (Tadasana) variation. **Photo #2**: Raised Hands Pose (Urdhva Hastasana). **Photo #3**: Tree Pose (Vriksasana). **Photo #4**: Warrior 1 Pose (Virabhadrasana I). **Photo #5**: Warrior 2 Pose (Virabhadrasana II). **Photo #6**: Archer Pose. **Photo #7**: Raised Arms Pose (Hasta Uttanasana). **Photo #8**: Standing Forward Bend (Uttanasana).

An example of the illustrations in the book is shown below:

Flow Chart of Posture Four
(Perform Movement 1 while walking forward.)

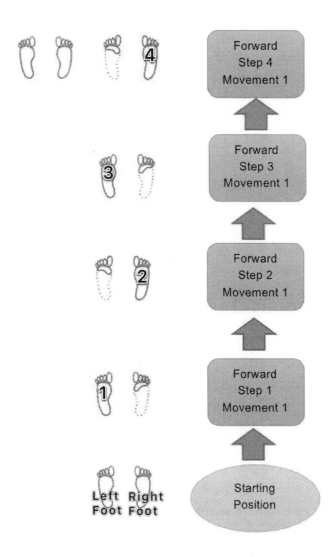

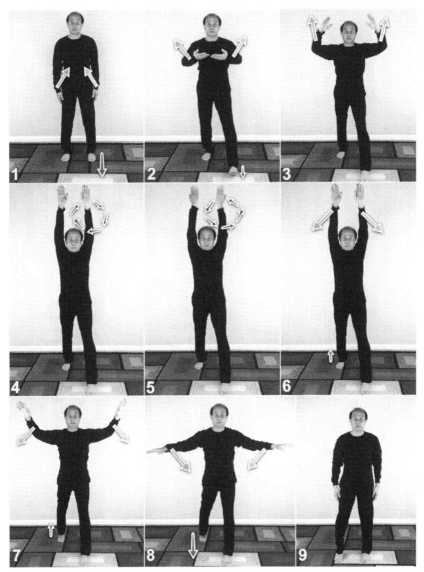

Figure 6-5A. Posture Four, the first step (front view).

A yoga pose, **Warrior 1 Pose**, is adopted in this posture (see Photos #4, #5, and #6).

Here you can see the unique feature of Yoga E Tai Chi: **Rotate the arms while staying in the pose** (see Photo #4 and Photo #5).

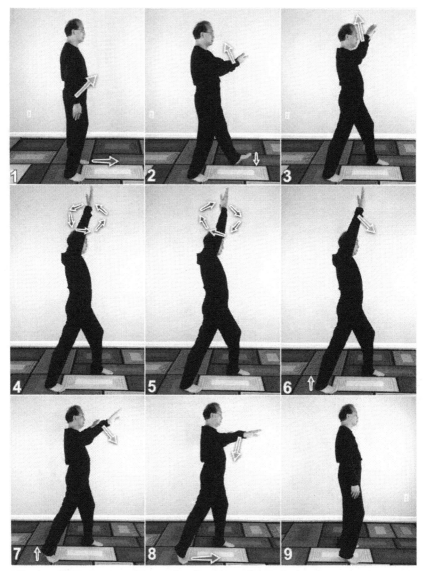

Figure 6-5B. Posture Four, the first step (lateral view).

A yoga pose, **Warrior 1 Pose**, is adopted in this posture (see Photos #4, #5, and #6).

Here you can see the unique feature of Yoga E Tai Chi: **Rotate the arms while staying in the pose** (see Photo #4 and Photo #5).

Introduction

Live life in harmony and balance. Avoid excesses. Even good things, pursued or attained without moderation, can become a source of misery and suffering.

—M. A. Soupios and Panos Mourdoukoutas
(Authors of *The Ten Golden Rules: Ancient Wisdom from the Greek Philosophers on Living the Good Life*) (Mourdoukoutas, 2012)

The first man that ever ran the marathon (around 26 miles) in 490 BC, Pheidippides, collapsed and died immediately after he reached his destination. Human beings were not designed for prolonged intensive aerobic exercises, and they have a storage of glycogen that provides energy only for 30 km/18-20 miles of running. For more details on this topic, see *Wikipedia: Marathon*. However, people hold more than five hundred marathons all over the world every year. Amateur marathon runners continue to be exposed to the marathon-induced harmful effects such as heart disorders, electrolyte imbalance, muscle and joint injuries, etc. Although I respect and admire the spirit of the marathon, I dislike the actual marathon running that poses health risks. Moderation in all things is the key.

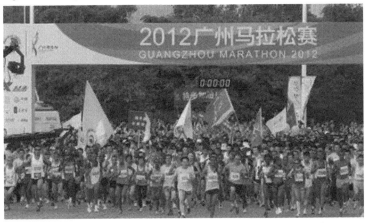

A recent article in Time magazine lists six simple exercises that have been proven effective in promoting health: walking, cycling, running, weight lifting, yoga, and tai chi (Oaklander, 2016).

Several patients of mine told me that their assisted living facilities provide tai chi training. However, most of my patients do not know what tai chi is. On the contrary, when asked if they know what yoga is, eight out of ten patients would say, "Yes, but it's difficult to do." It is estimated that more than 30 million adults in the US practice yoga (Yoga Journal, 2016). There are several yoga classes even in the small town where I practice.

Approximately 33,000 Americans died of opioid overdoses in 2015, according to the Center for Disease Control and Prevention. In the event of the opioid epidemic in the US, an author on Medscape even claims: **Opioid makers may have to teach physicians about yoga** (Lowes, 2017). Indeed, yoga has been proven to be helpful for pain management (Nahin, Boineau, Khalsa, Stussman, & Weber, 2016). Nevertheless, it is not realistic to require every physician who writes opioid prescriptions to learn yoga. Besides a higher risk of injury, yoga is probably more difficult to learn than tai chi. Especially, most of the yoga poses are too challenging for seniors or patients with chronic joint, back, or neck pain.

Unquestionably, yoga exercises have been proven to improve balance, flexibility, reduce stress and pain, etc. Still, if we exercise just for personal health, we do not have to stretch or twist our body parts extremely to achieve some "beautiful" poses or perform shoulder-stand/ headstand poses to "bring more blood to our brains."

I have done a lot of reading about yoga and practiced some safe poses during the past several years. I have found some standing yoga poses that are easy to learn and safe to practice after some modifications. Here, I have integrated these simple and safe yoga poses into E Tai Chi postures in order to achieve the stretching benefits that cannot be obtained by the relaxation in tai chi. I call this new yoga-tai chi combination exercise **"Yoga E Tai Chi"** or **"Yogetaichi."**

Yoga E Tai Chi is not the alternating performance of yoga and tai chi postures, but the yoga exercise that is integrated into E Tai Chi. It is the unified exercise of yoga and tai chi. Namely, each E Tai Chi posture includes some components of yoga. The partial arm extensions in tai chi and the full arm stretching in yoga coexist in each of the Yoga E Tai Chi postures.

All the yoga components in Yoga E Tai Chi are safe, even for older people. The Yoga E Tai Chi sequences maintain the basic features of tai chi: tranquility, slowness, relaxation, smoothness, and continuity. Yoga E Tai Chi is easy to learn and safe to practice. As with E Tai Chi, I hope you will live healthier and longer by practicing this simple and safe exercise, Yogetaichi, regularly.

I will keep all the basic information about E Tai Chi in this book. Hence, you can still learn Yoga-E Tai Chi by reading this book even if you do not know anything about E Tai Chi.

The following content is the introduction of my E Tai Chi Books. You can skip it if you have already read my E Tai Chi books.

Questions?

Why do I need to invent or create a new tai chi exercise since so many tai chi styles have already existed?

Why am I qualified to do this kind of work?

Why is E Tai Chi an invention?

When I entered the exam room, I found that Mr. Young, in his 40s, was standing with his hand holding the edge of the exam table painfully.

"Why are you standing, Mr. Young?" I asked.

"Doc, I am in trouble," he replied. "My back hurts like hell."

"What's happened? Lifting something heavy or a fall?"

"No. I went to a yoga class last night. I was okay then. However, when I woke up this morning, I cannot move my back at all. There is so much pain in the lower back that I cannot sit down. I feel less pain when standing up."

"I guess you have developed back injury probably due to overstretching during the yoga class."

"Please help me get rid of the pain, Doc."

The patient was one of the many yoga-induced injury cases I had encountered during the first few months after I started my new job in this town in 2013. For example, a woman complained of hip and groin pain after a few months' yoga exercises. A middle-aged man developed severe abdominal wall pain because of over-bending his body during a yoga session. A young yoga learner came in with a limping leg, complaining of leg pain with numbness of her foot and toes.

A couple of years ago, a patient of mine even collapsed while performing Yoga neck bending in the gym. She was sent to the ER by an ambulance. Fortunately, she had recovered completely without sequela.

Of course, many other patients come to see me because they suffer from a variety of musculoskeletal disorders after running, doing weightlifting, playing tennis or basketball or golf, etc. Unquestionably, all sports and physical exercises potentially cause injuries, especially in older people.

"I don't think you have a severe spinal injury," I said to Mr. Young after a physical exam. "I will prescribe some muscle relaxants and pain pills for you. Hopefully, you'll get better in a week or so."

"What next?"

"Stay away from yoga for a few weeks or forever."

"I like the mental exercise in yoga. What can I do in the future if I can't do yoga?"

"You can try tai chi. I think tai chi is another exercise that combines physical and mental workouts."

I showed him some tai chi performances on YouTube on the computer screen. I usually let my patients watch the 24-Form Simplified Tai Chi. Gao Jiamin's performance is always on the top list on YouTube.

"She is playing so smoothly and elegantly. She looks beautiful too," Mr. Young said.

"Sure, she is beautiful! However, you need to know she is a Chinese tai chi champion. You cannot imitate her long strides and high kicks. Those movements cause injuries as yoga does. The athletes do these for

26

a living like NBA players, who frequently check in to the orthopedic clinics and have their knees fixed during the off-season."

"I like it very much. How can I learn it?"

"You can buy a book with a DVD or watch YouTube videos."

"I got a tai chi video some years ago. But, it is too difficult to learn on my own. And I can't find a tai chi teacher around this area."

Many friends and patients told me that they bought tai chi books and DVDs in the past. However, they could not learn tai chi from those materials and gave it up eventually. All their tai chi books and DVDs are covered with dust on the bookshelf.

As the saying goes, "Learn to walk before you run." When it comes to tai chi learning, people tend to do the opposite. The most mysterious and unscientific thing I can think of about the contemporary tai chi is that almost all the tai chi forms have complicated beginning movements. Even in the Simplified 24 Form, you need to make a turn before you can go on to the next posture after finishing the **Commence** posture. What is the point of putting some complicated movements in the beginning postures of each tai chi sequence? These challenging starting postures scare away many potential tai chi learners.

Most of the tai chi books on the market are not easy to follow, especially without an instructor. Even some of the authors state in their books that one cannot learn tai chi by reading their books. Many tai chi books emphasize "**qi**" and "**dantian**," which have never been proved to be real scientifically. They are the old concepts of traditional Chinese Medicine, which are the primitive understanding of nature by the ancient people. The imaginary qi and dantian make tai chi more mysterious and harder to learn.

Furthermore, tai chi learners and practitioners tend to flex their knees too much. Over-flexion of knees may damage knee joints. The whole body weight is supported by only one leg in many postures. It is not safe for older people to perform those tai chi postures, which may cause joint injuries and falls.

As I work 10-12 hours daily and on some weekends, I cannot do any actual tai chi teaching. Over the past a few years, I have been thinking of designing a tai chi form everybody can learn without an instructor and perform anywhere, anytime without injury.

I have been showing E Tai Chi to some of my patients during office visits. They can learn it within five minutes. Some patients say that they forget it when they go home. Therefore, I decided to write a simple book on E Tai Chi so that everyone can use it at home. Finally, E Tai Chi has been created and introduced in the book, *E Tai Chi (The Basic Book)*.

Why am I qualified to write books about tai chi?

1. I have 45 years of experience in practicing Chinese martial arts.

2. I can practice all the popular tai chi forms: 24-Form, 48-Form, 42-Form, Yang, Wu, Hao (Wu), Chen, Sun, and Zhaobao styles. I can perform them not only traditionally from right to left but also in the opposite direction, from left to right. I have learned many prevalent qigong exercises.

3. I used to be a scientist with a Ph.D. degree and have a good knowledge of the structures and functions of the human body.

4. I am a practicing primary care physician, talking with patients about physical exercises daily and understanding how different sports affect them.

5. I came to the U.S. at the age of 31. I know how to read classic Chinese books on tai chi, Qigong, and traditional Chinese medicine (TCM). I am familiar with Chinese and English medical literature on tai chi studies.

6. I have collected and read more than one thousand tai chi and qigong books in both Chinese and English.

E Tai Chi is entirely distinct from the current tai chi styles. It is a style of simplicity and safety. Tai chi learners can learn E Tai Chi just by reading my book with accompanying videos. Moreover, it takes just hours or days to master it!

I believe **E Tai Chi** is the world's simplest and safest tai chi, which maintains the beauty of traditional tai chi and makes the best use of the health benefits of tai chi without injuries. E Tai Chi focuses on health benefits, and it does not care about so-called "tai chi fighting skills," which are misleading, impractical, and even dangerous.

E Tai Chi is simple because it consists of only **one** circular hand/arm movement and regular walking or standing. This single circular movement straightforwardly evolves into six basic hand/arm movements, which can be learned within two to three hours. Additionally, the hand/arm movements are symmetrical in most circumstances (except Movement 6, see Chapter 4 in the complete book). You can learn E Tai Chi without an instructor.

E Tai Chi is safe because it is composed of gentle hand/arm movements and regular walking or standing. You always face forward without making turns. Turning around can be dangerous to older people. Indeed, one can trip and fall even when taking a regular walk, particularly in the case of senior citizens. Nevertheless, this is life! We all need to be careful whenever we do something in our life.

It seems that no one has created a new style of tai chi since Wu style tai chi was designed eight decades ago. For example, the latest style of tai chi, Dongyue Taijiquan (东岳太极), was crafted by Professor Men Huifeng (门惠丰教授) in 2000 (Men 门, 2011). However, none of its movements or postures is newly designed. Namely, Dongyue Tai Chi is a sequence of tai chi forms that were chosen from the existing styles of tai chi and put together.

E Tai Chi is an invention because it is not a rearrangement or modifications of existing tai chi forms. It is a brand-new tai chi exercise system. Even though the six hand/arm movements in E Tai Chi look straightforward and familiar, five of them excluding **Cloud Hands** have never been seen before in all styles of tai chi. For example, all the current tai chi styles have Cloud Hands, but nobody has thought that Cloud Hands can be "reversed" to become **Reverse Cloud Hands**. Cloud Hands is executed **vertically** with **sideways walking** or standing in all the styles of tai chi. Has anyone imagined that Cloud Hands can be implemented **horizontally** or while walking **forward** or **backward**? In fact, you can take any direction you like when performing Cloud Hands in E Tai Chi. Furthermore, you can wave your hands in large or small circles because there is no strict rule in E Tai Chi. The only rule is easy, which means simple, safe, and gentle.

Even though these five movements are newly designed, they are derived from the essence of existing tai chi. Most importantly, they are easy to learn and safe to practice. Also, I get rid of unhealthy curved tai chi walk, jumps, kicks, Half Squat Stance (*pubu*), etc. I use regular walking or standing instead.

Thus, E Tai Chi is easy to learn, and one can practice it safely anywhere and anytime. Naturally, it takes weeks or months to improve your smoothness, continuity, and relaxation. However, you can build up your confidence right away by mastering E Tai Chi within minutes or hours. Since you can learn how to perform and enjoy it on the first day, you will practice it daily from that moment on and achieve its health benefits.

Chapter 1. Demystifying Tai Chi

《题西林壁》
横看成岭侧成峰，远近高低各不同。
不识庐山真面目，只缘身在此山中。

Written on the Wall at West Forest Temple
From the side, a whole range; from the end, a single peak:
Far, near, high, low, no two parts alike.
Why can't I tell the true shape of Lu-shan (Mount Lu)?
Because I myself am in the mountain.

—苏轼 (Su Shi, 1037-1101, Chinese poet)
Translated by Burton Watson

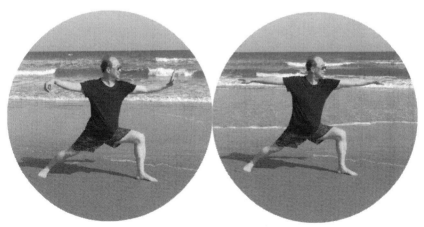

Left: Tai chi, Single Whip.
Right: Yoga, Warrior 2 Pose (Virabhadrasana II).

The above poem implies that *lookers-on see most of the game*. I have never had a formal tai chi teacher. I started to learn some tai chi postures from a co-worker more than 40 years ago when I was working at a printing factory in China. Since then, I have studied tai chi just from reading books, watching videotapes, videodisks, and observing people practice in the parks in China. Of course, I enjoy watching beautiful tai chi performances on YouTube and other Chinese video websites such as 56.com, youku.com, etc.

Because I do not claim to be a student or disciple of any tai chi master, I do not have the burden of keeping any one's style. Tai chi is simply my hobby, and I am good at it. As I do not teach or conduct research on tai chi for a living, I have no conflict of interests related to tai chi. What I have is science, modern medicine, and clinical experience. I create E Tai Chi and write a book about it for the purpose of helping my patients. Certainly, the book will benefit other people who are interested in simple and safe tai chi. That is to say, I am entirely an outsider to the field of tai chi. Hence, I am able to look at tai chi exercises from a different perspective.

Since yoga arrived in the west more than one hundred years ago, it has become more and more popular over the past several decades. Yoga classes are seen everywhere in the US and other parts of the world. There are thousands of yoga books on the markets, many of which were written by yoga scholars, master teachers, or gurus. Numerous yoga blogs exist on the Internet, and many thousands of yoga videos can be watched on YouTube. Thus, instead of opening up a lengthy discussion on yoga's history, health benefits, theories, and so on, I would like to make a concise comparison between tai chi and yoga that is pertinent to Yoga E Tai Chi. In the latter part of this chapter, I will describe tai chi exercises in detail.

Again, I have not learned any yoga pose from a yoga teacher or a master or a guru though I practice many yoga poses regularly and have benefited from them. Thus, it is likely that I can tell some truths about yoga as a yoga layman.

Tai Chi versus Yoga

Let's start with the **definitions** of yoga and tai chi:

"Yoga is a group of physical, mental, and spiritual practices or disciplines which originated in ancient India," as quoted from Wikipedia. (For more details on this topic, see _Wikipedia: Yoga._)

"Tai chi is an internal Chinese martial art practiced for both its defense training and its health benefits," as quoted from Wikipedia. (For more details on this topic, see _Wikipedia: Tai chi._)

Truly, yoga covers many more subjects than tai chi does, especially it puts more emphasis on its spiritual and philosophical aspects. Many yoga books describe that there are eight limbs of yoga: Yama (abstentions), Niyama (observances), Asana (postures), Pranayama (breathing), Pratyahara (abstraction), Dharana (concentration), Dhyana (meditation), and Samadhi (realization). For more details on this topic, see _Wikipedia: Yoga_. Traditionally, performing postures (asana) is considered to be only a part of these yoga disciplines or a preparation for meditation. Indeed, yoga masters or gurus pursue enlightenment, samadhi, and the like.

Nevertheless, whenever I use the term "yoga," I mean yoga asana (postures), including simple breathing and meditation only. I am convinced that there are many better ways of learning personal morality or good hygiene other than through yoga.

Since tai chi originated as a martial art, the most famous treatise of tai chi, _The Taijiquan Treatise_ by Wang Zongyue, focuses on how to keep balance and to throw an opponent away. (See an English translation of the Taijiquan Treatise by Louis Swaim (Fu (Author) & Swaim (Translator), 2012)). Tai chi is not only a martial art but also a competitive sport in modern times. Numerous tai chi tournaments are held each year all over the world. There are countless tai chi champions. You have not heard any yoga champion though there are numerous yoga master teachers and gurus. You may learn yoga from certified yoga teachers while anyone can teach tai chi exercises.

In the west or in modern times, yoga is primarily an exercise routine signified by pose performance, which often includes breathing training and meditation. Most people practice tai chi or yoga for the purpose of improving health. In this book, I concentrate on the health aspects of yoga and tai chi. Honestly, I do not care too much about combat applications in tai chi or spiritual enlightenment in yoga.

History

It is still debatable how long yoga has come into existence. Definitely, yoga has a much longer history than tai chi does. Tai chi was probably created in China about 800 years ago, while yoga originating in India is thought to have existed for 2500 to 5000 years. Over the past several decades, both yoga and tai chi have become known to the world and gained more and more popularity. It is estimated that there are approximately 36 million yoga practitioners in the US in 2016 (Yoga Journal, 2016), and 3.5 million people practice tai chi in the US in 2015 (Statista, n.d.). American yoga practitioners spent $16.8 billion in 2016 on yoga classes, clothing, equipment, and accessories (Yoga Journal, 2016). Since yoga is a big business with a peculiar origin, there have been multiple scandals surrounding yoga gurus over the years (Broad, 2012) (Grant, 2015) (Herrington, 2017). It is possible that similar scandals involving tai chi masters are uncommon because I have performed some Google searches using the term "tai chi scandals" and have not found one comparable case yet.

The theories of energy centers and channels are used in both yoga and tai chi. Apparently, there are more chakras in yoga, while tai chi masters emphasize only one "energy" center, dantian. Qi in tai chi and prana in yoga are thought to travel or circulate through these centers and channels. The channel system is called nadi in yoga and meridians in tai chi. All these centers, channels, and qi/prana were imagined by the ancient people thousands of years ago. These concepts or structures are related to the human nervous system in modern science. For decades, yoga practitioners, including yoga gurus, have already used their knowledge of modern neuroscience, anatomy, physiology, psychology, etc. to explain or describe yoga theories or phenomena. For instance, Swami Rama, a yoga guru, used a lot of scientific concepts to elucidate his yogic views (Rama, 1992) (Rama, 2002) (Rama, 2009). Nevertheless, it seems to me that the old concepts such as the meridian system, yin/yang, dantian, etc. continue to be the theoretical foundation of tai chi or qigong nowadays (Liu & Qiang, 2013) (Yang, 2015). Undoubtedly, more scientific studies have been carried out on yoga than on tai chi according to my search on the PubMed website entering the term "yoga" or "tai chi."

Even more schools or styles of yoga have been created than tai chi styles. A new yoga book lists more than 50 styles of yoga (Wei & Groves, 2017) while there are only six major tai chi styles: Chen, Yang, Wu, Hao, Sun, and Zhaobao styles. I have not known any government-designed yoga exercise yet. However, 24-Form, 48-Form, 42-Form, and 88-Form Tai Chi were developed by the Chinese government sports committee several decades ago. Later on, the Competition Forms of Yang, Chen, Wu, Hao (Wu), and Sun styles have come into being through the Chinese government support.

Over recent years, the Indian government has been actively promoting yoga (Huffpost, 2017), and the United Nations General Assembly declared June 21st as the **International Day of Yoga** in 2014. Similarly, **World Tai Chi and Qigong Day** takes place on the last Saturday of April each year across the globe since 1999. For more details on the **International Day of Yoga** and **World Tai Chi and Qigong Day**, please refer to *Wikipedia*. At the end of the day, I still believe that yoga or tai chi should be regarded as one of the many exercises that improve personal health, and that either of them or both together cannot save the world.

Health benefits

Both yoga and tai chi help improve balance, strength, and flexibility, calm your mind, and reduce stress. In yoga, each pose or a group of poses are thought to improve one specific disease or several diseases (McCall, 2007) (Fishman, 2014). On the contrary, no one has claimed to treat any disease by performing a particular tai chi posture.

Like other alternative medicines, yoga and tai chi have turned out to be able to improve some chronic medical conditions that are related to the musculoskeletal system, pain, and stress. In most circumstances, they are not superior to modern medicine even in the treatment of those disorders such as chronic musculoskeletal pain, depression, anxiety, hypertension, migraine, etc. For example, a recent study indicates that yoga is as effective as physical therapy, but not better than education in the treatment of chronic low back pain (Saper, Lemaster, Delitto, & al, 2017). Certainly, they cannot treat infections like HIV and Hepatitis C, or cancers. However, they promote health and well-being and provide alternative ways to treat some chronic diseases.

You'd better not think that yoga or tai chi can solve all your health problems. Living healthy and long relies on many things such as good genes, a stable society, a safe environment, an optimal health care system, advanced medical care, and a healthy lifestyle. A healthy lifestyle includes a healthy diet, adequate sleep, regular and moderate exercises, without bad behaviors such as smoking, heavy drinking, and drug abuse. Exercises like yoga and tai chi are merely one of the various components of a healthy lifestyle.

In regard to medical applications (i.e., treatment of a specific disease), yoga or tai chi may be used as adjunctive therapy. Recently, the Australian Government published a review of alternative medicine. It suggests that there is **no** clear evidence that all the 17 natural therapies, including yoga and tai chi, have therapeutic efficacy (Australian Government Department of Health, 2015). Absolutely, yoga or tai chi is still like a horse, not a modern transportation vehicle. Apparently, *"modern transportation provides us with cars, planes, ships, and trains which carry us much farther away at higher speeds. You will surely get to your destination almost all the time…You cannot go too far by riding a horse, and horses cannot carry thousands of people to work every day as subways do. People can fall from horses and become paralyzed,"* as quoted from my memoir (Li, 2015).

Injuries

Yoga asana is a strenuous exercise that requires persistent stretching and staying in poses. Performing yoga poses tend to place your body in unusual positions for extended periods of time. Consequently, yoga can cause various injuries, including sprains, strains, joint dislocations, bone fractures, ligamentous or muscle tears, and even strokes (Broad, 2012). It leads to many emergency room visits yearly in the U.S. Even some yoga teachers suffer themselves. Some breathing exercises lead to extreme hypoventilation or hyperventilation, which can have adverse consequences. Yoga meditations have been reported to cause mental disorders such as psychosis. (Penman, Cohen, Stevens, & Jackson, 2012) (Broad, 2012).

In contrast, tai chi is much more gentle, relaxed, and smooth with fewer adverse effects (Wayne, et al., 2014). You seldom take the awkward postures that are not used in everyday life. Since tai chi is a dynamic exercise requiring walking, it can cause knee pain or injury, as described in the latter part of the chapter. Surely, **E Tai Chi** is the safest tai chi with few or no side effects.

Almost all the tai chi books do not elucidate physical injuries. For example, Professor Deyin Li, probably the most famous tai chi teacher in China, does not explain in his book what injuries tai chi can cause (Li 李德印, 2003). On the contrary, most of the recent yoga books bring up these issues. For instance, the author of *Yoga as Medicine* states in his book (McCall, 2007) that he himself developed thoracic outlet syndrome, which led to numbness and tingling in his right hand, because of performing Headstand, Shoulder Stand, and Plow Pose. Recent studies showed that approximately 20-30 percent of yoga class attendees had suffered adverse side effects (Matsushita & Oka, 2015) (Cramer, Ostermann, & Dobos, 2017).

In a newly published yoga book, *The Harvard Medical School guide to yoga* (An excellent yoga book. Wei & Groves, 2017), though the authors have devoted a whole chapter to discussing how to prevent yoga injuries, they state, "In a 2015 review of yoga studies from 1975 to 2014, **yoga was found to be as safe as walking or stretching exercises**, even for people with a wide variety of health issues." It seems to me that walking is perhaps the safest exercise or sport on earth. By using common sense, you can conclude that the statement "*yoga is as safe as walking*" cannot be true. Obviously, as mentioned in the reference the above authors cited (Cramer, et al., 2015), fewer than one-third of the analyzed randomized controlled trials of yoga (94 out of 301) included the topic of yoga-induced injuries.

However, later on, the authors write (Wei & Groves, 2017), "Poses such as Plow, Shoulder Stand, and Headstand pose can be particularly **risky** for your head and neck area. We don't teach these poses in our book for this very reason…" Actually, Headstand was considered to be "one of the most important Yogic asana" or "the king of all asana" by the yoga guru, B. K. S. Iyengar (Iyengar, 1995).

The "supreme" pose for meditation, Lotus Pose, can easily cause knee/ankle pain or injuries (Cole, 2007). There is no scientific evidence that putting your feet on top of your thighs in Lotus Pose makes people live healthier and longer. In addition, I don't think that meditating in Lotus Pose or in any seated position for a long time is healthy because too much sitting can shorten your life (Biswas, et al., 2015) (Diaz, et al., 2017).

Lifting your foot above or behind the head in yoga is simply a form of entertainment like Olympic gymnastics, which has nothing to do with health improvement or spiritual growth. In the same way, striking the ground forcefully with one's foot in tai chi (e.g., in Chen style) plays no role in fighting opponents, but leads to knee pain or injury. Remember that the health benefits of yoga and tai chi come from the gentle, regular exercises of your body, not from those risky "beautiful poses." Moderation is always the key.

Difficulty.

Tai chi and yoga highlight both physical and mental exercises. As I will discuss thoroughly in the next section, it is difficult to learn traditional tai chi. When compared with tai chi, yoga is even harder to learn. Not only coming into some yoga poses are challenging but coming out of them requires extreme care.

Generally speaking, tai chi has only fewer than 40 postures. Even though there are more postures in Chen style tai chi, I do not consider Chen style as a typical tai chi. It seems to me that new tai chi postures or styles had not appeared for 80 years until E Tai Chi was created and published by the author in 2016. There are only ten simple and easy postures in E Tai Chi.

In contrast, many more yoga poses have been created. For example, B. K. S. Iyengar demonstrated more than 200 poses in his famous book, *Light on Yoga: The Bible of Modern Yoga* (Iyengar, 1995). More and more yoga poses have come into being over the years though many of them are hard to perform, challenging, and even dangerous.

In terms of breathing, most tai chi books written in Chinese barely touch upon this subject. For example, Li Deyin, the most famous tai chi teacher in China, writes only two paragraphs about the breathing principles in his 500-page tai chi book (Li 李德印, 2003). Meditation is seldom involved in tai chi teaching though tai chi masters emphasize that your mind should lead or conduct your hand/arm movements.

Numerous breathing and meditation techniques are used in yoga. Many books specifically on these subjects have been published. (Rama, 2009) (Rama, 1992) (Saraswati, 2016). It takes days, months, or longer to master these techniques, some of which, such as Breath of Fire, may be dangerous and harmful. I am sure that only simplicity can make an exercise, a sport, a game, or even everything in life great.

Performing Postures

When it comes to performing postures, both yoga and tai chi emphasize relaxation, especially relaxing the shoulders. In tai chi, you need to "drop" (gently flex) your elbows and "settle" (gently extend) your wrists. Namely, your arms are never at full stretch. Even though you may take an extremely brief pause (less than half a second) at the conclusion of a tai chi posture, the transitions between postures are smooth. Tai chi postures are performed slowly and continuously one after another.

Arms are fully extended and stretched out in many yoga poses. You hold a pose for a much longer period of time, which can be several breaths or even minutes. The activity of persistent yoga stretching provides a specific therapeutic effect that cannot be achieved with tai chi. In yoga sequence exercises, you can execute poses sequentially, but not in a flowing motion like tai chi.

In tai chi, you never touch the ground with your hands or sit on the floor. Your body weight is always supported by your legs. Especially, there is no inversion posture in tai chi. You need to keep the torso straight without bending and hold the head upright. And you need to contain the chest. In other words, you should not thrust your chest forward. Each tai chi posture is supposed to have some combat applications. In fact, you can kick with feet, push with palms, and punch with fists.

In yoga, you use not only your legs, but also hands/arms, shoulders, back, or/and head to support the body weight. You need to open your chest up on many occasions. You can bend forward, backward, and to the side. You can even arch your back and lock the joints. But, you don't see any movement implying fighting in a yoga pose.

Since you need to balance your body with your arms supporting the body weight in many yoga poses, yoga practice offers an intensive strength-training workout for your upper extremities and core muscles. When you are in unusual acrobatic positions, you can stretch out the ligaments and muscles that you cannot do in tai chi. These strenuous exercises in yoga incur a higher risk of injury than those gentle ones in tai chi. Ultimately, Yoga E Tai Chi is the simplest and safest yoga-tai chi combination exercise.

Summary of Comparison between Tai Chi and Yoga

	Tai Chi	Yoga
Origin	China.	India.
Dated	Around 800 years.	2500-5000 years.
Definition/Goal	A martial art for defense and health.	Physical and mental training for health and spiritual growth.
Participants in the US	3.5 million.	36 million.
Competition Sport	Yes.	No.
Certified Teachers	No.	Yes.
Styles	Fewer than ten.	Dozens.
Theory	Qi, dantian, and the meridian system.	Prana, chakras, and nadi.
Health Benefits	Balance, strength, flexibility, pain reduction, and stress relief.	Similar to tai chi. But it is assumed to treat many more diseases.
Practice	Usually, in an open space.	On a yoga mat.
Injuries	Mainly knee pain or injury.	A variety of injuries. More serious.
Difficulty to Learn	Yes.	Yes, more than tai chi.
Number of Postures	Fewer than 40.	More than 100.

Posture or Pose Execution	Smoothly, gently, and continuously.	Not in a flowing manner.
Walking	Yes.	No.
Sitting	No.	Yes.
Stretching Fully	No.	Yes.
Holding Poses	No.	Yes.
Inversion/Bending	No.	Yes.
Bearing the Body Weight	By legs only.	By arms, shoulders, legs, back, and head.
Kicking/pushing/jumping.	Yes.	No.
Physical Training	Legs and waist.	Arms, legs, and core muscles.
Breathing/Meditation	Subtle.	Strongly emphasized. Numerous methods.
Body-Mind Exercises	More mind training.	Both.

Further Readings on Yoga:

For health professionals: *Principles and Practice of Yoga in Health Care.* (Khalsa, Cohen, Mcall, & Telles, 2016) (538 pages)

For general yoga practitioners: *The Harvard Medical School Guide to Yoga: 8 Weeks to Strength, Awareness, and Flexibility.* (Wei & Groves, 2017) (336 pages)

For the knowledge of yoga scientific foundation: *A 21st-Century Yogasanalia: Celebrating the Integration of Yoga, Science, and Medicine.* (Robin, 2017) (3117 pages).

For the history of yoga: *The Yoga Tradition: Its History, Literature, Philosophy, and Practice.* (Feuerstein, 2013) (550 pages)

Further Readings on Tai Chi:

The Harvard Medical School Guide to Tai Chi: 12 Weeks to a Healthy Body, Strong Heart, and Sharp Mind. (Wayne & Fuerst, 2013) (353 pages).

The following sections of this chapter have appeared in my E Tai Chi Books. You can skip them if you have already read my E Tai Chi books.

What Is Tai Chi?

Tai chi is an abbreviation of Tai Chi Chuan or Taijiquan. **Tai Chi (Taiji, 太极)** means the origin of the universe, "supreme ultimate," in Chinese, which is not related to martial arts. Here **Chuan** or **Quan** (拳) means "fist or boxing" in Chinese. I will use tai chi in most circumstances in this book because I dislike anything implying "fighting." (For more details on this topic, see *Wikipedia: Tai chi.*)

Tai chi, one type of Chinese martial arts, is characterized by its tranquility, slowness, relaxation, smoothness, and continuity. It is a combination of physical and mental exercises. Chinese martial arts (wushu，武术) have been existing for thousands of years. They are merely individual or personal fighting skills and have nothing to do with real wars in Chinese history. Although tai chi masters emphasize its fighting techniques, tai chi has never been proved to be a practical fighting skill even in one to one fighting, and never played any role in battlefields. A famous Chinese general, Qi Jiguang (戚继光, 1528－1588), wrote several hundred years ago, "Learning a martial art is for enhancing physical fitness only, not for fighting in battlefields." Numerous anecdotes tell that prominent tai chi masters could throw away opponents without bodily contact. Yet, no one has ever been able to demonstrate this type of technique in front of a camera.

In the West, boxing is purely a fighting sport. On the contrary, tai chi, the most popular Chinese martial art, has been incorporated into Chinese culture, sports, and entertainment. There have been dozens of martial art movies that depict the mysterious, "superior" tai chi fighting. Overemphasizing its combat aspect will be misleading, impractical, and even dangerous in the 21st century.

Many tai chi books claim that tai chi is a great treasure of China's cultural heritage. However, most Chinese people did not know the existence of tai chi until the Chinese government started to promote it in the 1950s and 1960s. Tai chi has never played any significant role in eliminating diseases, promoting population health, bringing prosperity, and repelling invaders in Chinese history.

In summary, tai chi can be considered to be one of the many exercises or sports that improve **personal** health. Nevertheless, tai chi is unique because it emphasizes both physical and mental training. Most importantly, tai chi is a safe exercise or sport (Wayne, et al., 2014). It has been scientifically proven to have many health benefits (Hempel, et al., 2014). It not only helps to improve some medical disorders but also cultivates the sensation of feeling good through its slow, smooth, relaxed movements. This gentle and comfortable exercise is particularly suitable for older people.

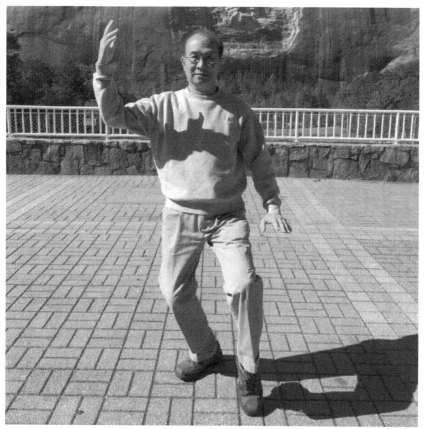

White Crane Spread Its Wings in traditional Tai Chi.

A Brief History of Tai Chi

The origin of tai chi is still controversial. However, Zhang Sanfeng (张三丰, in the 12th century?), a legendary Taoist, is commonly considered as the creator of tai chi. But there were several Taoists known as Zhang Sanfeng. Tai chi was initially practiced by Taoists or monks secretly. Most books state that a businessman named Wang Zhongyue (王宗岳, in the 15th Century?) happened to learn tai chi from someone (a Taoist?). Then he taught tai chi techniques to Zhang Fa (张发, in the 15th century?), who lived and learned tai chi in Wang's home for seven years. Zhang Fa started to teach tai chi when he came back to his hometown, Wen County, Henan Province, China. It is debatable who Zhang Fa's first student was. At least, it has been well documented that people in the area started to practice tai chi four hundred years ago. (For more details on this topic, see *Wikipedia: Tai chi*.)

Until the late 1800s, tai chi had been practiced for several hundred years only by small groups of individuals like monks, some martial art teachers, and their dedicated students. The majority of tai chi practitioners and learners lived in Henan Province, China, during that time. The story tells that Yang Lushan (杨露禅, 1799-1872) went to Chen Village, Henan Province, and stayed there many years learning tai chi. Yang Lushan returned home and then went to Beijing, the capital city of China, to teach tai chi. Since then, tai chi has spread out to other parts of China over the next 100 years and then to many other countries over the past 50-60 years.

Tai chi is hard to learn. There is a saying, "It takes ten years to master tai chi." Some great teachers, such as Yang Chengfu (杨澄甫, 1883-1936) had tried to simplify tai chi and created Yang style tai chi, which is easier to learn. Tai chi masters have created many different styles of tai chi. There are six most popular tai chi styles as follows:

Yang style tai chi is the most popular one that was simplified and standardized by Yang Chengfu (杨澄甫).

Chen style tai chi is commonly considered as the oldest tai chi originated in Chen Village, Henan Province. The creator of Yang style tai chi lived and studied tai chi in the village.

Zhaobao style tai chi has existed for a long time like Chen style tai chi. Some people think that Chen style tai chi is derived from Zhaobao tai chi, which is the original tai chi created by Zhang Sanfeng, the legendary creator of tai chi.

The other prevalent styles include Wu, Hao (Wu), and Sun. They were all rooted in Yang style. (For more details on this topic, see *Wikipedia: Tai chi*.)

Finally, the Chinese government organized tai chi experts to design the 24-Form Simplified Tai Chi in 1955. The government had also trained thousands of instructors to teach 24-From for free in China. As a result, millions of people can practice 24-Form in China. Since then, 48-Form, 42-Form, 88-Form Yang Tai Chi have been designed by the government sports committee. Later on, the Competition Forms of Yang, Chen, Wu, Hao (Wu), and Sun styles have come into being.

All these government-designed tai chi exercises are simply the rearrangements and minor modifications of the traditional tai chi forms. Nonetheless, their movements, forms, or postures have been standardized and scientifically designed to be more symmetrical and become easier to learn. Many tai chi teachers have immigrated or traveled to other countries and taught tai chi for the past several decades. It is estimated that there are more than one hundred million tai chi practitioners and learners all over the world.

The Health Benefits of Tai Chi

Tai chi is a unique exercise that combines physical and mental training. Any moderate and safe exercise can make you live better and longer (Lear, Gasevic, & Hu, 2016). Simplicity and moderation are everything in life. One should never do anything excessively. You do not have to exert yourself to the utmost or stretch your body immensely to achieve the health effect of an exercise or sport. Practicing tai chi can offer some specific health benefits without serious injuries (Hempel, et al., 2014).

In my opinion, tai chi can promote health mainly in two areas, reducing stress and improve musculoskeletal functions. Stress is related to almost all common chronic diseases, including coronary artery disease, hypertension, stroke, diabetes, mental diseases such as depression, anxiety, etc. Slow and relaxing tai chi movements help people become more relaxed and distracted from their stresses. As the stress level is lowered, these chronic disorders such as hypertension and depression can be improved or even eliminated.

Tai chi has been proven to alleviate musculoskeletal pain and stiffness, improve gait balance, reduce falls in senior citizens or patients with Parkinson's disease, and speed up recovery from a stroke. A recent review by VA has summarized the evidence of tai chi potential benefits in hypertension, depression, fall, balance confidence, osteoarthritis, pain, COPD, muscle strength, and cognitive performance (Hempel, et al., 2014).

Although practicing tai chi provides many health benefits, **tai chi is not a panacea**. It does not cure HIV, treat Ebola, or get rid of polio. I can guarantee that it does not cure or prevent hair loss. Yang Chengpu (杨澄甫, the creator of Yang style tai chi), was bald in his 40s according to his photos. If you want to look at his picture, see *Wikipedia: Tai chi*. So am I. Certainly, tai chi cannot cure cancer. But it may improve the quality of life in patients with cancer (Zeng, Luo, Xie, Huang, & Cheng, 2014).

This book is intended to show you how to practice E Tai Chi. If you want to know more about the health benefits of tai chi, you can refer to Wikipedia and the references in this book or read the book by Dr. Peter Wayne (Wayne & Fuerst, 2013).

The Shortcomings of Existing Tai Chi

Although the modern tai chi forms have their standardized movements and postures, they are only the rearrangement and minor modification of the traditional tai chi styles and cannot get rid of the shortcomings of the traditional tai chi, for example, they are still difficult to learn, especially for non-Chinese.

All the tai chi styles except the 24-Form Tai Chi have some complicated beginning movements including **Grasp the Bird's Tail** or **Lazy about Tying Coat**. Particularly, even the **Commencing** postures in Chen style and Zhaobao style tai chi are difficult to learn. I am not sure if tai chi masters intended to drive tai chi learners away or to impress their students. Anyhow, tai chi students have to spend weeks or months studying these several movements even if they do not quit.

All the tai chi books on the market are difficult to follow, esp. without an instructor. Even some of the authors state in their books that one cannot learn tai chi by reading their books. Some of the tai chi movements are too challenging for ordinary people to learn, e.g., **Lotus Kicks** and **Half Squat Stance** in almost all the tai chi styles. How many regular tai chi learners can perform **Dragon Dives to the Ground** (雀地龙) in Chen style tai chi? This posture is not only difficult to learn but

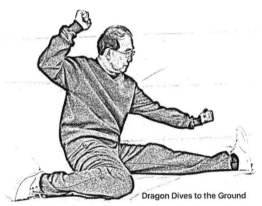

Dragon Dives to the Ground

also harmful to joints. Furthermore, it cannot be a practical fighting technique either.

Many tai chi books pay too much attention to fighting applications when teaching tai chi movements. Some books state that you cannot

48

master real tai chi if you do not know the martial applications of each posture. Few people learn tai chi for the purpose of fighting or even self-defense. That will make it harder to learn tai chi. In my opinion, you will grasp the real meaning of tai chi when you have completely forgotten its fighting techniques and power. Then you will become peaceful and relaxed and achieve its health benefits.

It has not been reported that amateur tai chi learners suffer a stroke or severe neck/back injuries because of practicing tai chi. Here, I am not talking about professional tai chi athletes. They jump or kick as high as possible and squat as low as possible. Remember that you do not imitate the leg movements of tai chi masters on DVD or YouTube. They are professionals, athletes, and champions, who do these performances for a living, but not for health purposes. They entertain us with those beautiful and challenging acrobatic movements, which have nothing to do with promoting health.

Although tai chi does not cause serious adverse effects such as fatal or life-threatening events, it can induce overuse injury to joints. The most common disorder caused by tai chi is knee pain or injury. Interestingly, in the west, some studies indicate that practicing tai chi can alleviate knee pain (Wang, et al., 2016) (Yan, et al., 2013) (Nahin, Boineau, Khalsa, Stussman, & Weber, 2016). The majority of the tai chi studies did not mention adverse effects caused by practicing tai chi. (Wayne, et al., 2014). In a recent study on the effect of tai chi on knee osteoarthritis, the authors reported no serious adverse events such as fatal, life-threatening, incapacitating events, hospitalizations, etc. without mentioning anything about worsening knee pain (Wang, et al., 2016). Surprisingly, it seems that all the participants in the tai chi and physical therapy groups had achieved beneficial effects on their knees (Wang, et al., 2016). Nevertheless, no medical treatment modality is free of adverse effects. In my clinical practice, my patients tell me from time to time that knee treatments with physical therapy, steroid injection, or even knee surgery make their knee pain worse.

On the contrary, tai chi induced knee pain and injury are very common in China (Zhu, et al., 2011). A recent survey found that more than 50 percent of tai chi practitioners reported knee pain after practicing tai chi (Yuan 苑显英, 2014). Tai chi-induced knee pain has become a hot topic in the tai chi community and got its nickname "Tai Chi Knee (太极膝)." Numerous studies and articles on this subject have been published in China. You can do a google search if you are interested in this issue.

Many tai chi students tend to over-flex their knee joints because a lot of tai chi teachers and professional athletes practice tai chi this way. You can watch their performances on YouTube. For example, the image of **Outdoor practice in Beijing's Temple of Heaven** on Wikipedia shows a tai chi practitioner (the man wearing a white shirt and black pants in the center of the picture), whose front knee is over-flexed and protrudes over the toes even though his stance is high. (For more details on this topic, see *Wikipedia: Tai chi.*)

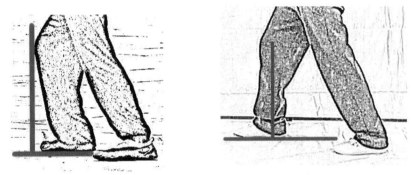

Figure 1-4A. Knee flexion in a bow stance. Left: Incorrect Stance. The front knee protrudes over the toes of the foot. Right: Correct Stance. Ideally, the front leg should be perpendicular to the foot or ground.

Taking a low stance and long strides will place even more strain on the knees and other joints, leading to not only knee but also ankle and hip injuries. Life is contradictory. Delicious food is usually unhealthy. Similarly, the long stride and low stance look beautiful but are harmful to joints, especially knee joints.

In many styles of existing tai chi including 24-Form, practitioners cannot keep their knees aligned with the tips of their feet when making turns and rotating the torso because of some of the unhealthy tai chi postures. The abnormal twisting of the knees can easily cause knee injuries. For example, when you perform the first **Parting the Wild Horse's Mane** posture after finishing **Commencing** in 24-Form, you must step out to the left with your left foot while turning the torso left at the same time. Because the supporting knee (the right knee) is not in line with the tip of the foot, knee pain or injury is likely to occur. See **Figure 1-4B**.

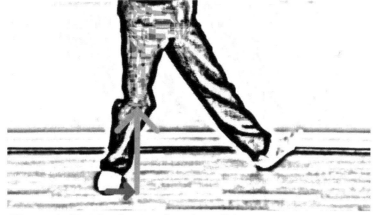

Figure 1-4B. The first Parting the Wild Horse's Mane posture in 24 Form Tai Chi. The supporting knee (the right knee) is not aligned with the tip of the foot.

In many postures of traditional tai chi, people are not supposed to move their steps straightforward, but in a curved route. First, they need

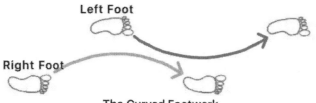

Left Foot

Right Foot

The Curved Footwork

to rotate their legs to turn their torso and shift the body weight. Secondly, they move their swinging foot close to the standing foot and then shift it back to the original side. The rotation of the legs may twist the knee and ankle joints, and the supporting leg will carry the whole-body weight for an extended time. As a result, the knee and ankle joints can easily get hurt. The curved walking is especially unsafe for older people.

When it comes to "fighting," no real fighter would like to use tai chi footwork or curved walking in an actual fight, as has been demonstrated in modern-day fighting competitions such as tai chi sanshou, boxing, karate, and any other martial arts. All fighters adopt a natural stance with mildly flexed knee joints. Furthermore, there is no evidence that curved walking provides more health benefits than regular walking. In addition, no martial art master takes a horse stance or a bow stance when carrying out a fight even in a movie.

For millions of years, human beings have used natural walking to carry out most of their activities. They have walked out of Africa and reached every corner of the world. Walking on foot differentiates us from other animals. Walking is the most natural way to move around. We need to keep walking for almost all our lives.

Why do we need a tai chi step or footwork that is harmful to joints? Is it because my teacher's teachers or my ancestors did this way? Sun style tai chi has the safest way to walk because the rear foot follows the front foot closely without loading the body weight on one leg for an extended period of time. Naturally, when people stand and wait in line, they tend to use one foot to support the body weight, the other foot lightly touching the ground for balance only. Unfortunately, the most popular tai chi, 24 Form, preserves the curved footwork.

All the traditional styles of tai chi except Chen style are not aerobic exercises and do not increase upper extremity strength effectively even though all of them provide a lot of lower-extremity training. Of course, too much weight-bearing would destroy the smoothness and relaxation of tai chi. Tai chi is not a panacea. You need to do weight workouts if you want to build up muscles. Alternatively, you can speed up metabolism by running, playing tennis, etc.

Any moderate and safe physical exercises have health benefits and can make you live better and longer. Tai chi is simply one of them. Most importantly, you exercise moderately, safely, and regularly.

Chapter 2. The Characteristics of E Tai Chi & Yoga E Tai Chi

Everything should be made as simple as possible, but not simpler.
—Albert Einstein (1879 – 1955, German-born theoretical physicist)

Simple can be harder than complex: You have to work hard to get your thinking clean to make it simple. But it's worth it in the end because once you get there, you can move mountains.
—Steve Jobs (1955-2011, American entrepreneur and inventor)

"The proverb says you do not need more than enough of anything. I have learned that moderation is the key to everything in life and medicine. One should never do anything excessively. Too much exercise may hurt your joints and even your heart, and excess eating can cause many diseases, including obesity and diabetes. Eating right and exercising judiciously will make you live better and longer." (Quoted from my book, ***Life and Medicine***.)

E Tai Chi is a symbol of moderation and simplicity.

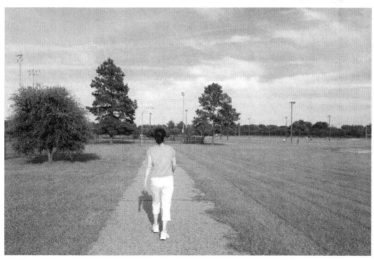

Taking a walk in the park.

E Tai Chi

*This section of the chapter has appeared in my E Tai Chi Books. If you have already read my E Tai Chi books, you can skip it and go on to the next section: **Yoga E Tai Chi**.*

These days, **E**-anything is a cool name, such as e-mail, e-book, e-commerce, and even e-medicine. "E" in **E Tai Chi** is an abbreviation of "**Easy** or **Ease**," not "electronic." "Easy" or "ease" means simple, gentle, and comfortable. **E Tai Chi** is a style of simplicity, gentleness, and comfort.

I would like to compare E Tai Chi to **Metformin** (antidiabetic medication). Metformin, the treatment base for type 2 diabetes, is the most widely prescribed antidiabetic in the world. It has also been used in many other conditions, including polycystic ovarian syndrome, prevention of diabetes, weight control, adjunct cancer therapy, and even dementia.

Metformin originated from French Lilac. (See details in the section of Chapter 5: Diabetes-Metformin as Herbal Medicine in my book, *Life and Medicine*.) (Li, 2015) Scientists started to extract the active ingredients from French lilac in the 1800s. However, all those extracts that could lower blood sugar level in animals and humans turned out to be too toxic for clinical use. One of the extracts was scientifically modified to become a useful and safe drug, Metformin.

For the same reason, even though having health benefits, traditional tai chi has many shortcomings as described above. E Tai Chi is scientifically extracted and developed from the traditional tai chi. Through cautious modification and redesign, tai chi has become simple, easy to learn, and causes less or no injury from practicing it (with few or no adverse side effects).

E Tai Chi is a newly invented style of tai chi, which is entirely different from the current tai chi styles. E Tai Chi emphasizes simplicity, safety, and health benefits. It is for personal health only and has nothing to do with fighting or even self-defense. There are only six hand/arm movements in E Tai Chi. Except for **Cloud Hands** that exists in all the tai chi styles, the remaining five movements look straightforward, but they are completely newly designed. Furthermore, the typical tai chi walk, catwalk, has replaced by regular walking or slowed natural walking. Therefore, I call it an invention.

In addition to maintaining all the health benefits of traditional tai chi, E Tai Chi has the following advantages, which can be summarized as the **Five S's**: **Simplicity, Science, Safety, Strength,** and **Serenity.**

Simplicity. As I mentioned previously, I have condensed all the current tai chi movements into only **one** circular movement. In biology, a cell is the basic structure of living organisms, the simplest unit of life except for viruses. Similarly, E Tai Chi is the tai chi exercise at the cellular level. Therefore, it cannot be simplified anymore if you want to maintain the essential characteristics of tai chi.

There are numerous hand/arm movements, stances, and kicks in traditional tai chi. Even in the book about standardized tai chi, Professor Li Deyin (李德印教授) introduces 33 hand/arm movements, 10 stances, 14 ways of walking, and 6 types of kicking (Li 李德印, 2003). In E Tai Chi, you perform **six** hand movements, **five** stances, and **three** ways of normal walking without kicking, squatting, or making turns.

In E Tai Chi, the single circular hand/arm movement gives rise to the **six** basic movements readily. The symmetry of its movements makes it easy to learn and remember. You can learn E Tai Chi without an instructor. Movements 1, 2, and 3 are so easy that everybody can learn them within minutes. If you perform them while standing or walking naturally, then you can say you have learned E Tai Chi.

Unlike traditional tai chi forms, Posture One is the simplest form at the beginning of the basic E Tai Chi sequence. The following Postures are as simple as Posture One. Movement 4 in E Tai Chi is the traditional **Cloud Hands (Wave Hands like Clouds)**. Although it is one of the most beautiful tai chi postures, most of the tai chi books describe it in a very complicated way. I do not think any tai chi beginner can learn how to perform Cloud Hands by reading those books. Here I can summarize Cloud Hands in **one** sentence: **sequentially circle your hands in front of you while walking sideways or standing.**

Therefore, it takes only two to three hours to master the basic E Tai Chi postures. You have finished the learning process in E Tai Chi if you do not want to go any further. Late on, what you need to do is to practice, perfect, and enjoy it.

Science. E Tai Chi is a complete brand-new training system, which is scientifically designed according to the principles of simplicity, safety, and efficacy. It is not based on unscientific concepts such as Yin/Yang, meridians, Five Elements, imaginary organs, and so on.

As mentioned earlier, knee pain is a major injury due to practicing tai chi. A higher degree of knee flexion during tai chi practicing poses an increased risk of suffering tai chi-induced knee pain (Yuan 苑显英, 2014).

The normal gait cycle consists of eight phases: initial contact, loading response, midstance, terminal stance, preswing, initial swing, midswing, and terminal swing. The knee joints sustain the most weight load during the loading and midstance phases. The maximum knee flexion during the loading and midstance phases is 15-20 degrees (University of Washington) (Dicharry, 2010) (Rose, n.d.). The average walking step length is about 26.4 inches (67 cm) for women and 30 inches (76 cm) for men (The United States Department of Veterans Affairs).

Since walking is the safest and most efficient exercise for human beings, I have tried to make the walking exercise in E Tai Chi as close to the natural walking as possible. I adopt the 15-20-degree flexion of knee joints in E Tai Chi **Routine Stance** (see Chapter 3) after reviewing a lot of scientific research on walking gait and tai chi exercises. However, the degree of knee flexion will be increased spontaneously when you practice slow normal walking in E Tai Chi sequences. I propose that the flexion of the knees should not be over 20-30 degrees, and the length of each step should be within 30 inches (76 cm) in order to prevent knee injuries. See **Figure 2-1A**. Also, the knee should always be kept in line with the tip of the foot.

You can practice E Tai Chi anywhere and anytime. You can perform the hand/arm movements in any direction, horizontally, diagonally, and vertically. The circular hand movements can be expanded and shrunk to achieve different exercise effects. Even though I illustrate the core principles of performing E Tai Chi, there is no strict rule. The rule is that you are doing right as long as you feel natural, comfortable, and painless. E Tai Chi should not cause more pain even if you have knee pain before practicing it. If it is the case, you need to keep adjusting your stance with less flexion of knee joints and shorter steps until your knee pain returns to its baseline level. Alternatively, just walk naturally as usual.

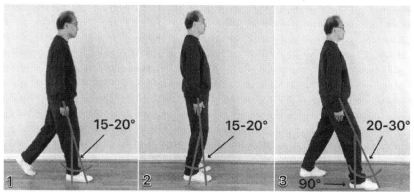

Figure 2-1A. Knee flexion during normal walking, in Routine Stance, and during slowing walking in E Tai Chi sequences.

Photo #1: Normal walking during the loading response phase. The knee joint reaches 15-20 degrees of peak flexion. The step length is about 2 feet (60 cm), which is comfortable for me.

Photo #2: Routine Stance. This stance is taken all the time when practicing E Tai Chi sequences.

Photo #3: Slow walking in E Tai Chi sequences. The degree of knee flexion should be kept within 30 degrees. The lower leg should be perpendicular to the ground, and the knee should be aligned with the tip of the foot.

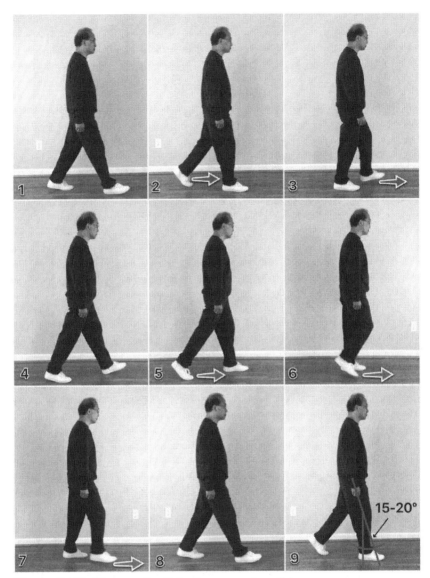

Figure 2-1B. Phases of gait during normal walking.

Key points for **Figure 2-1B**.

Photo #1: **Initial Contact.** The right foot is moving forward with the right heel touching the ground.

Photo #2: **Loading Response**. Shift your body weight to the right leg with the entire right foot contacting the ground. Lift the left heel up and get ready to step forward with the left foot.

Photo #3: **Midstance**. The left foot is swinging forward.

Photo #4: **Terminal Stance**. The left heel touches the ground. Gradually shift the body weight to the left leg.

Photo #5: **Preswing**. The body weight has moved entirely to the left leg with the right heel raised off the ground. You are ready to step forward with the right foot.

Photo #6: **Initial Swing**. The right foot is swinging forward and passing the left foot.

Photo #7: **Midswing**. The right foot continues to move forward.

Photo #8 (= Photo #1): **Terminal Swing**. The right heel comes in contact with the ground. Now you can repeat the same cycle of normal forward-walking.

Photo #9: The same as **Photo #2 (Loading Response)**. The peak flexion of the knee.

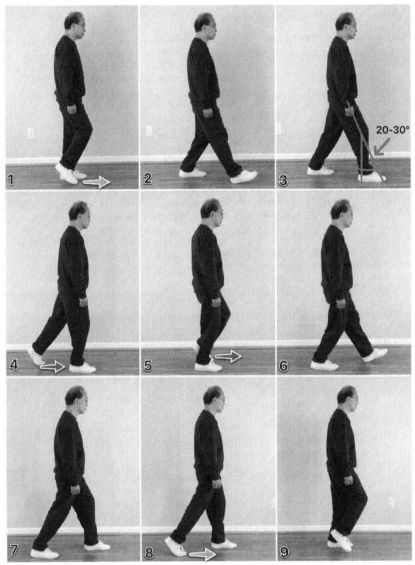

Figure 2-1C. Slow forward walking in E Tai Chi sequences.

Key points for **Figure 2-1C**.

Photo #1: This is **Transitional Stance**: one of the legs (the left leg in the figure) is supporting the body weight while the toes of the other leg (here the right leg) gently touch the ground to maintain balance.

Photo #2: Step forward with the right foot. The right heel comes in contact with the ground.

Photo #3: Gradually shift the body weight to the right leg. Now, you are in **Bow Stance**: your front knee (here the right knee) is mildly flexed with the back leg (here the left leg) straight.

You should use the rear leg to push the body forward so that the front lower leg forms a 90-degree angle relative to the front foot or the ground. This is a standard **bow stance** in Chinese martial arts. When **you drive the body forward by the rear leg**, the front knee joint will not be over-flexed. That is the most critical measurement to prevent knee injuries. This principle applies to all the forward movements.

Photo #4: As the body weight is completely transferred to the right leg, the left heel comes off the ground. You are ready to swing the left leg forward.

Photo #5: The left leg swings forward until it becomes parallel to the right leg. The toes of the left foot gently touch the ground. Now you are back in **Transitional Stance**.

Photo #6: Step forward with the left foot with the left heel hitting the ground.

Photo #7: Gradually shift the weight to the left leg. Again, you are in **Bow Stance**: your left knee (the front knee) is mildly flexed with the right leg (the back leg) straight.

Photo #8: As the body weight is entirely shifted to the left leg, the right heel comes off the ground. You are ready to swing the right leg forward.

Photo #9: The right leg is swinging forward, and your right foot becomes parallel to the left foot (the front foot). The toes of the right foot (the back foot) gently touch the ground while the left foot continues to support the body. Now you are back in **Transitional Stance**.

Safety. The typical tai chi walk, the curved walk, has been replaced by natural walking or slowed natural walking in E Tai Chi. You always face forward without making turns, squatting, or kicking.

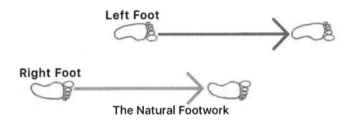

The footwork in natural walking and E Tai Chi.

Most postures in all the current tai chi styles involve a slow forward walking. The knee joint will sustain a lot of strain during walking forward because the position of the front knee is far away from the midline of the body. In contrast, the chance of getting knee injuries will be much lower during walking sideways or backward as the position of the knees is very close to the midline. Additionally, walking sideways requires much less flexion of the knee joints than walking forward. Because you walk sideways in most of the E Tai Chi postures, you can avoid over-flexion of the knees and maintain optimal knee-foot alignment. You may not feel pain when doing the sidestepping workout if you suffer from knee pain before practicing tai chi. Walking sideways not only poses a low risk of knee injuries but also offers some specific therapeutic potential (see below).

Since E Tai Chi involves only gentle hand/arm movements and regular standing or walking, it should not incur more risks than a person's usual daily activities do. When you practice the E Tai Chi sequences, you will slow down your walking pace. On the one hand, the slow execution of tai chi can provide a good workout on lower extremities and relax your mind. On the other hand, it may strain your knee joints if you are a beginner or at an advanced age. Therefore, I have designed **Transitional Stance** to solve this problem. Namely, you can take a break by placing your swinging foot parallel to the standing foot during the midswing phase of the gait cycle. See **Figure 2-1C**.

All these safety designs will minimize injuries induced by tai chi exercises. You can practice E Tai Chi safely anywhere, anytime, and in any position (sitting, standing, walking, or even lying). Thanks to its gentle arm/hand movements and regular standing or walking, E Tai Chi is safe, especially for older people.

Strength. In the E Tai Chi sequence, the majority of the postures involve sideways walking. E Tai Chi provides an efficient physical workout because walking sideways consumes over three times more energy than walking forward (Handford & Srinivasan, 2014). Older individuals have a reduced ability to take side steps to avoid obstacles (Gilchrist, 1998). They are at higher risk of falling laterally and suffering a hip fracture (Maki & Mcllroy, 2006). Sideway training is used in rehabilitation in patients with stroke, brain injuries, or Parkinson's disease (Kim & Kim, 2014) (Bryant, Workman, Hou, Henson, & York, 2016). Therefore, sideways walking exercise will help prevent falls in older adults.

According to a recent study, the most common knee symptom among tai chi practitioners is lateral knee pain, which is consistent with iliotibial band syndrome (Yuan 苑 显 英 , 2014). Strengthening exercises, including sidestepping, are an effective treatment for iliotibial band syndrome. Sidestep training has been used in physical therapy to alleviate back pain and pain disorders affecting lower extremities (ACE Physical Therapy and Sports Medicine Institute, 2015). Therefore, the emphasis on walking sideways in E Tai Chi not only decreases the risk of getting tai chi induced knee pain or injury but helps relieve knee pain due to other causes such as patellofemoral pain syndrome.

You can rise up onto tiptoes when practicing the advanced E Tai Chi. Standing or walking on your tiptoes can help improve balance, calf strength, posture, and ankle function.

E Tai Chi can be combined with a strength-training workout if you wear some weights on your wrists and ankles. You can make E Tai Chi an aerobic exercise by speeding up the hand/arm movements.

Serenity. E Tai Chi combines with qigong, a specific Chinese breathing/meditation exercise like yoga. You can easily coordinate your breathing with hand movements because all the hand/arm movements are symmetrical.

E Tai Chi relaxes your body, reduces stress, promotes physical fitness, and cultivates the sensation of feeling good.

You do not have to face the west or the east when you practice E Tai Chi or Yoga E Tai Chi. There is no scientific evidence that facing the east is healthier than facing the west, the north, or the south. In E Tai Chi or Yoga E Tai Chi, you can walk in any direction or even walk circularly.

You can create your own E Tai Chi sequence by using the six basic hand movements and different ways of walking or standing. These hand /arm movements can be easily transformed further into any movements of existing tai chi styles. Therefore, E Tai Chi has laid a solid foundation for you if you wish to pursue traditional tai chi forms in the future.

Yoga E Tai Chi

Yoga E Tai Chi is a yoga-tai chi combination exercise that is developed on the basis of E Tai Chi. Not only does it maintain all the characteristics of E Tai Chi, but it contains the yoga elements that are simple and safe. Definitely, it preserves the five S's of E Tai Chi: **Simplicity, Science, Safety, Strength,** and **Serenity.** Here, I will explain these features again but in more detail.

Simplicity.

In the basic Yoga E Tai Chi, I have adopted only eight standing yoga poses (see **Figure 2-2A**):

Mountain Pose (Tadasana) variation that is integrated into Sideward Movement 2;

Raised Hands Pose (Urdhva Hastasana) into Upward Movement 1;

Tree Pose into Balance Postures;

Warrior 1 Pose (Virabhadrasana I) into Forward Movement 1;

Warrior 2 Pose (Virabhadrasana II) into Sideward Movement 1;

Archer Pose into Sideward Movement 3;

Raised Arms Pose (Hasta Uttanasana) into Backward Movement 2;

Standing Forward Bend (Uttanasana) into Downward Movement 2. (How to perform Movements 1, 2, and 3 will be found in Chapter 4.)

The above yoga poses are simple and effective. They can be practiced safely after having been modified and integrated into E Tai Chi. The hand/arm movements in yoga and tai chi have been condensed to only **ONE** circular movement. In Yoga E Tai Chi, you always use the same circular hand movement to get into and out of a pose. Please see the following example, **Posture One** (see **Figure 2-2B**).

Photos #4, #5, and **#6** in **Figure 2-2B** show how you come into the pose. Lower your hands until your arms are fully extended and stretched out at shoulder level with the palms facing down and your head facing leftward. What you achieve is the Warrior 2-like pose. **Photos #7, #8,** and **#9** show how you come out of the pose. Circle your hands down and return them to your sides. Then you are ready to perform the next pose.

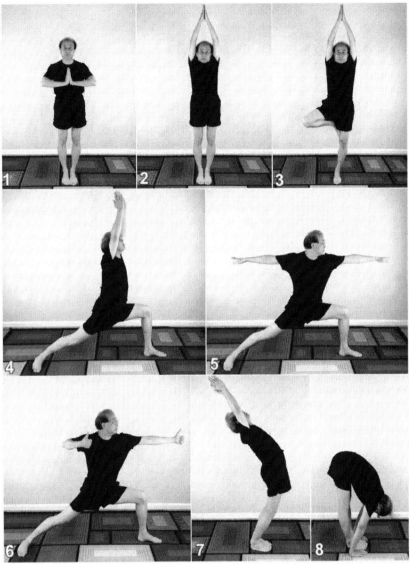

Figure 2-2A. Eight yoga poses are adopted in the basic Yoga E Tai Chi. **Photo #1**: Mountain Pose (Tadasana) variation. **Photo #2**: Raised Hands Pose (Urdhva Hastasana). **Photo #3**: Tree Pose (Vriksasana). **Photo #4**: Warrior 1 Pose (Virabhadrasana I). **Photo #5**: Warrior 2 Pose (Virabhadrasana II). **Photo #6**: Archer Pose. **Photo #7**: Raised Arms Pose (Hasta Uttanasana). **Photo #8**: Standing Forward Bend (Uttanasana).

The simple circular hand movement can easily get you into the pose and get out of the pose. Once you have learned a pose, you will never forget how to perform it. You are always in a standing or walking position without holding the bodyweight with your hands, elbows, shoulders, or head. You do not need yoga uniforms, yoga mats, or other supporting materials. You can practice Yoga E Tai Chi anywhere and anytime. Especially, you can practice these simple stretching/holding exercises in the workplace every 30 to 60 minutes because prolonged sitting is bad for health (Biswas, et al., 2015) (Diaz, et al., 2017). You may not need to go to a yoga class anymore because you can always watch my video demonstrations on YouTube or in the e-book.

You practice the same hand/arm movements and sequences as in E Tai Chi. If you have mastered E Tai Chi, then you can pick up Yoga E Tai Chi within an hour. You can still learn Yoga E Tai Chi by reading this book and the accompanying videos if you do not know E Tai Chi at all. It probably takes a few hours to master the basic Yoga E Tai Chi postures without knowledge of E Tai Chi (please see the study plan).

Science.

Yoga E Tai Chi is a yoga-tai chi fitness routine that is developed on the basis of E Tai Chi. In other words, E Tai Chi assimilates the typical elements of yoga: holding poses and stretching fully. Thus, you can find both yoga and tai chi components in each of the Yoga E Tai Chi postures. **Distinctively, the arms keep rotating even when they are fully extended and stretched out.** See **Photos #6** and **#7** in **Figure 2-2B**. This unique feature that can **only be seen** in Yoga E Tai Chi enhances the efficacy of yoga stretching, maintains the continuity of tai chi postures, and synchronizes your breathing with the hand movements seamlessly. You can repeat the arm rotating movements as many times as you like, depending on how long you want to stay in a pose.

As demonstrated in **Figure 2-2B**, you practice tai chi first by circling your arms up and then get into a yoga pose easily. After coming into the yoga pose, you hold it and rotate your arms at the same time with breathing coordination. The arm rotating movements are perfectly coordinated with a breathing exercise. Later on, you finish the posture by circling your arms down and returning your hands to your sides. The whole yoga-tai chi posture is performed smoothly and gently without abrupt interruption of movements. Consequently, the sequence exercises are smooth and continuous.

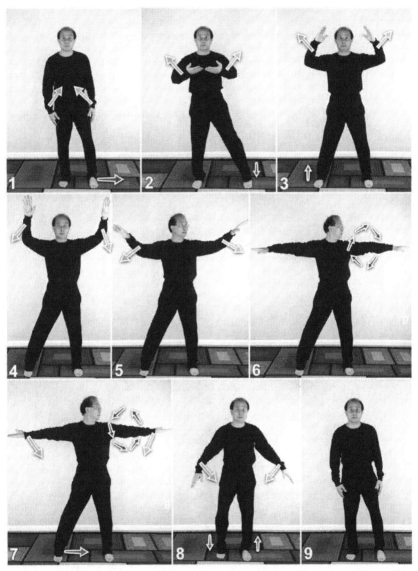

Figure 2-2B: Posture One: walk sideways leftward and perform Sideward Movement 1.

Key points for **Figure 2-2B**.

Photo #1: **Routine Stance** to **Transitional Stance**. Stand with feet shoulder-width apart. The knees are flexed at 10-20 degrees. Shift your body weight to the right leg. Lift the left heel up and get ready to step out.

Photo #2: Take a step out leftward with your left foot when you are raising your hands along the midline. The toes of the left foot are touching the ground. **Inhale** while raising the hands.

Photo #3: Gradually shift your body weight to the left leg while continuing circling your hands up. At this moment, the body weight is evenly distributed between your legs.

Photo #4: As your hands are raised overhead, the body weight has been completely moved to the left leg, and the right heel comes off the ground. Your palms face forward.

Photo #5: Exhale while lowering the hands without moving your feet. Gradually turn your head toward the left.

Photo #6: Your arms are fully extended and stretched out at shoulder level with the palms facing down and your head facing leftward. You can hold this pose for one breath or as long as you like. This pose looks like **Warrior 2 Pose** in yoga except that your stance is higher, and your right heel is off the ground.

Next, **inhale** and slowly rotate your arms to turn the palms upward (supinate) while keeping stretching out your arms.

Photo #7: The palms have been turned to face upward. Hereafter, **exhale,** and circle your hands down while turning your palms downward.

Photo #8: Move the right foot closer to the left foot while dropping your hands. In the meanwhile, pronate your arms so that your palms face downward. The toes of the right foot are touching the ground at this moment.

Photo #9: Gradually shift your bodyweight back to the right leg as your hands return to your sides. At this moment, you are back to **Transitional Stance** with the right leg supporting the weight and are ready to step out with the left foot again.

As we know, holding a pose can not only improve muscle strength and stamina but increase the body-mind connection and build confidence. Yoga E Tai Chi maintains the characteristics of tai chi exercise: relaxation, smoothness, and continuity. At the same time, it assimilates the main features of yoga: holding poses and stretching fully without their shortcomings, such as being difficult to learn, causing joint injuries, etc.

Since tai chi is defined as a martial art, each tai chi posture is supposed to have some combat applications. So, you need to keep the head upright and the torso straight without bending. You need to contain the chest. Namely, you should not thrust your chest forward. Consequently, you cannot perform effective neck turning, chest expanding, and back bending exercises in tai chi.

In Yoga E Tai Chi, you can bend forward, backward, and to the sides (see **Figure 2-2C**). Moreover, you can look upward, downward, and to the sides with rotating the torso (see **Figure 2-2D**). Not only can you expand and stretch your chest, but also you can stand on one foot to perform balance postures (see **Figure 2-2E**). Thus, Yoga-E Tai Chi provides a comprehensive workout for the neck, chest, and back, shoulders, and legs.

Traditional yoga is a static exercise because you do not walk around while performing yoga poses. Practicing yoga components while walking in Yoga E Tai Chi enhances the efficacy of yoga workout. Especially, walking sideways in the sequence practice can strengthen leg muscles, improve balance, and reduce lower-extremity joint pain. You can execute the hand/arm movements vertically, horizontally, in any circular manner, and with any combination of vertical and horizontal performances.

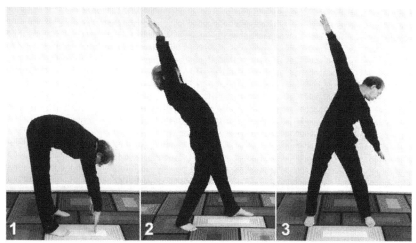

Figure 2-2C. Bending exercises in Yoga E Tai Chi. **Photo #1**: Bending forward (Downward Movement 2). **Photo #2**: Bending backward (Backward Movement 2). **Photo #3**: Bending to the side with gentle rotation of the torso (Sideward Movement 5, which will be described in the advanced book.)

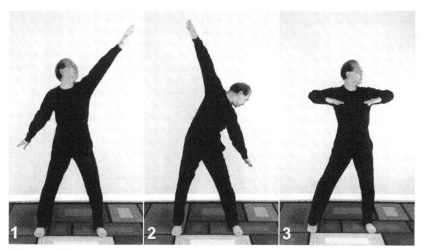

Figure 2-2D. Neck exercises in Yoga E Tai Chi. **Photo #1**: Look upward (Sideward Movement 4, which will be described in the advanced book.) **Photo #2**: Look downward with gentle rotation of the torso (Sideward Movement 5). **Photo #3**: Look to the side while expanding and stretching the chest (Sideward Movement 2).

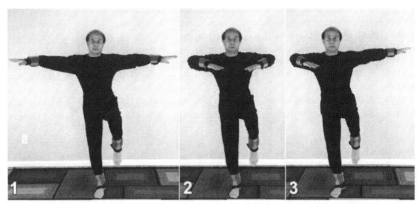

Figure 2-2E. Stand on one foot with weights on hands and ankles. Expand and open the chest.

Safety.

As with E Tai Chi, you stand, walk naturally, or walk at a slower pace when practicing Yoga E Tai Chi. You do not make turns, squat, or kick. There is no extreme bending and twisting. Because you walk sideways in most of the postures, you can avoid over-flexion of the knees and maintain optimal knee-foot alignment.

Only several safe and effective standing yoga poses, which have been modified, are included. It is especially suitable for older people because a lot of floor or balance poses in yoga may be unsafe for them. Especially, I don't recommend any advanced inversion poses (such as handstand, headstand, and shoulder stand), where your body is upside down and supported by your head, hands, shoulders, or forearms. These upside-down poses can easily cause injuries. All the postures in Yoga E Tai Chi are safe if you practice them gently and comfortably. However, you need to be cautious and do some modifications if necessary when performing downward Movement 2 and Backward Movement 2. See **Figure 2-2F** and **Figure 2-2G**.

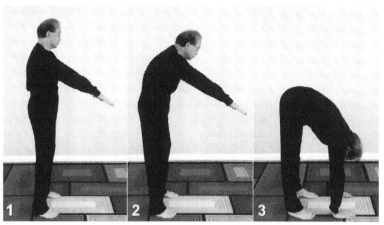

Figure 2-2F. Variations of Forward Bending in Downward Movement 2. Do not bend at all (**Photo #1**) or Bend forward to a lesser degree (**Photo #2**) if you have certain health conditions like back or neck pain/injury, dizziness, glaucoma, and cardiovascular diseases. **Photo #3**: Touch your palms on the floor and keep your knees straight if you have good flexibility.

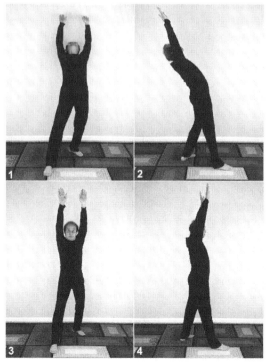

Figure 2-2G. Variations of Backward Bending in Backward Movement 2.

Photos #1 and **#2**: Bend backward as far as you feel comfortable.

Photos #3 and **#4**: Bend backward to a lesser degree or do not bend at all if you have certain health conditions like back or neck pain/injury, dizziness, and cardiovascular diseases.

Any exercise or sport, including natural walking, can cause injuries if you do not do it carefully. You should stretch, rotate, or bend your joints, neck, and back gently, slowly, and comfortably. On a daily basis, we need to bend down to pick up something like performing Downward Movement 2 or reach up to get something like performing Backward Movement 2. Although, as described above, these two postures need to be performed carefully, they should not pose a greater risk of injury than people's normal daily activities do.

Serenity.

Breathing exercises have been proven to be able to soothe one's mind. However, the hand movements in both traditional tai chi and yoga poses were not designed to coordinate with breathing workout. For example, most of the breathing exercises in yoga are carried out in a seated still position. Also, some yoga breathing exercises cause extreme hypoventilation or hyperventilation, which can lead to adverse consequences. Yoga meditations have been reported to cause mental disorders such as psychosis (Broad, 2012).

Even though breathing exercises are emphasized in Yoga E Tai Chi, only **ONE** safe exercise technique is recommended: conscious natural breathing coordinated with hand/arm movements. This technique can be mastered and practiced easily because most of the hand/arm movements are symmetrical. You can easily coordinate your hand movements and your breathing, as demonstrated in **Figure 2-2B**:

Inhale while raising the hands (see **Photos #1, #2,** and **#3**);

Exhale while lowering the hands (see **Photos #4** and **#5**);

Inhale while turning the palms upward (supinate) (see **Photo #6**);

Exhale while dropping the hands and turning the palms downward (pronate) (see **Photos #7** and **#8**).

You can always follow the simple rule: inhale when raising your hands (or the leading hand) and exhale when lowering your hands (or the leading hand). Similarly, breathe in when turning the palms upward/forward and breathe out when turning the palms downward/backward.

The breathing in Yoga E Tai Chi is natural, conscious, gentle, and effective. You do not need to think about which nostril is used or which muscles in the body are contracted in Yoga E Tai Chi. I am sure that you will achieve most of the health benefits of tai chi/yoga training by this simple and safe breathing method. Please read the section on **Breathing** in the next chapter for more details.

Strength.

In the Yoga E Tai Chi sequences, the majority of the postures involve walking sideways. Yoga E Tai Chi provides an efficient physical workout because sideways walking consumes over three times more energy than forward walking. You can tone up your muscles by performing Yoga E Tai Chi with weights on your wrists and ankles (see **Figure 2-2E**). Moreover, you may even turn Yoga E Tai Chi into an aerobic exercise if you practice it at a fast pace.

Just as it's true with E Tai Chi, you can create your own Yoga E Tai Chi sequence by using the six basic hand movements and different ways of walking or standing. Yoga E Tai Chi relaxes your body, reduces stress, promotes physical fitness, and cultivates the sensation of feeling good. Since Yoga E Tai Chi is simple and safe, you can easily incorporate it into your day to day life. You can practice it safely and effectively anywhere and anytime alone or with your friends or family members. You will save a lot of time and money because you do not need to go to a yoga class anymore.

A proposed study plan

Basic Yoga E Tai Chi (It takes three to five hours to learn it.)
Learn the hand/arm movements: Movements 1, 2, and 3 (5-15 minutes).

Learn the standing postures.
a. Upward/Forward Postures with Movement 1 (15-30 minutes);
b. Sideward Postures with Movements 1, 2, and 3 (15-30 minutes);
c. Downward/Backward Postures with Movement 2 (15-30 minutes);
d. Balance Postures with Movements 1, 2, and 3 (15-30 minutes).

Learn the basic walking sequence (five postures plus Starting and Closing Postures).

Starting Posture: Upward Movement 1;

Posture One: Sideward Movement 1 while walking sideways (15-30 minutes);

Posture Two: Sideward Movement 2 while walking sideways (15-30 minutes);

Posture Three: Sideward Movement 3 while walking sideways (15-30 minutes);

Posture Four: Forward Movement 1 while walking forward (15-30 minutes;

Posture Five: Backward Movement 2 while walking backward (15-30 minutes);

Closing Posture: Downward Movement 2.

The following contents will be covered in Yoga E Tai Chi (The Advanced Book).

Intermediate Yoga E Tai Chi (one to two days)

1. Learn the hand/arm Movements 1 to 6.

2. Learn the standing postures with Movements 1 to 6.

3. Learn the intermediate walking sequence (ten postures plus Starting and Closing Postures).

Advanced Yoga E Tai Chi (one to two days)

1. All above.

2. Learn the advanced walking sequence. The same ten postures as in the intermediate sequence are performed but in a different way. Namely, vertical and horizontal hand/arm movements are performed alternately with rotating the torso.

Chapter 3. The Basics of E Tai Chi (also Used in Yoga E Tai Chi)

千里之行始于足下。

A journey of a thousand miles must begin with the first step.

—老子 (Lao Tzu, 571 B.C., Chinese philosopher)

行路难

行路难，行路难。多歧路，今安在？
长风破浪会有时，直挂云帆济沧海！

Hard is the way, hard is the way.
Don't go astray! Whither today.
A time will come to ride the wind and cleave the waves,
I'll set my cloudlike sail to cross the sea which raves.
—李白 (Li Bai, 701—762, Chinese Poet)
Translated by 许渊冲 (Xu Yuanchong)

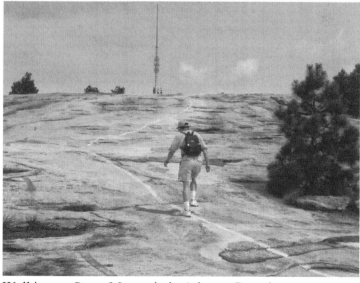

Walking up Stone Mountain in Atlanta, Georgia.

*All the basic stances, footwork, breathing methods, and hand/arm movements used in E Tai Chi are adopted and implemented in Yoga E Tai Chi. Therefore, the contents of Chapters 3 and 4 have been included in the E Tai Chi books. You can skip these two chapters if you have learned E Tai Chi. **But you need to read the section about breathing, which has been expanded.***

There are numerous hand/arm movements, stances, and kicks in traditional tai chi. For example, in his book about standardized tai chi, Professor Li Deyin (李德印教授) teaches 33 hand/arm movements, 10 stances, 14 ways of walking, and 6 types of kicking (Li 李德印, 2003). It scares away many potential tai chi learners.

In E Tai Chi, there are only five stances, three ways of walking, and six hand/arm movements without kicking, jumping, and squatting. You can turn your palms in any direction. You are doing it right if you do not feel awkward and can perform comfortably. After you have learned the basics in this chapter and the next chapter, you will go on to grasp E Tai Chi without difficulty and succeed in becoming a master of E Tai Chi.

Stances

There are many stances in traditional tai chi, including the Simplified 24-Form. Many of these different stances provide no proven health benefits and may even hurt your joints. There are only five simple stances in E Tai Chi as follows:

Stance One: **Normal Standing**.

Stance Two: **Routine Stance**.

Stance Three: **Transitional Stance**.

Stance Four: **Empty Stance**.

Stance Five: **Bow Stance**.

Stance One: **Normal Standing**

Stand naturally in a relaxed state with your feet shoulder-width apart and with knees straight. Feet are naturally placed with toes pointed forward. Keep your head upright and your eyes looking forward. Relax your shoulders. Hang your hands and arms loosely at your sides. See **Figure 3-1A**.

All the tai chi books emphasize that the tip of the tongue should touch the roof of the mouth behind the upper teeth. It was believed that you could connect the imaginary "circulation" to let "qi (energy)" move around the body. You do not need to think about the position of your tongue in E Tai Chi. Anything natural and comfortable is fine.

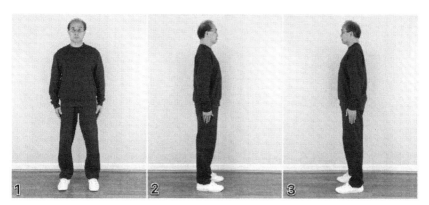

Figure 3-1A. Normal standing.

79

Stance Two: **Routine Stance**

Stand or move with the knees flexed at 10-20 degrees. Feet are naturally placed with toes pointed forward. See **Figure 3-1B**. When carrying out regular walking, you typically bend your knee joints to the same extent. If normal walking does not hurt you, then this angle of flexion will be appropriate. You use this stance most of the time when practicing E Tai Chi sequences.

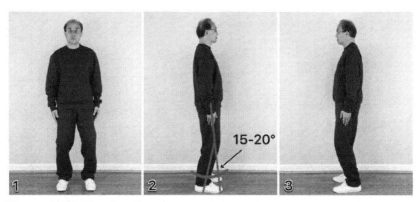

Figure 3-1B. Routine Stance.

The Important Point

Bend your knees to a lesser degree or do not flex them at all if you feel uncomfortable or pain in this stance.

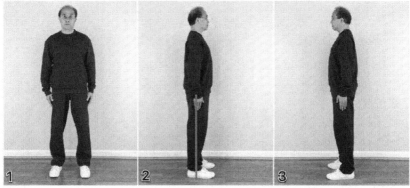

Figure 3-1Bb. Routine Stance without knee flexion (normal standing).

Stance Three: Transitional Stance

Stand with one foot (the right foot in the figure) supporting the body weight. Another foot (here the left foot) with the heel off the ground is gently placed parallel to the supporting foot. The toes of both feet are pointed forward. The knee (here the right knee) of the supporting leg is bent at 10-20 degrees. See **Figure 3-1C**. This stance is the typical posture in which we stand relaxedly when carrying on a casual conversation or waiting in line.

You can use this stance to do all the transitions from one posture to another posture when walking forward, backward, and sideways. This stance is unique and never seen in other styles of tai chi. It differs from the follow-up stance in Sun and Hao style tai chi. The back foot is positioned behind the front foot in Sun and Hao styles.

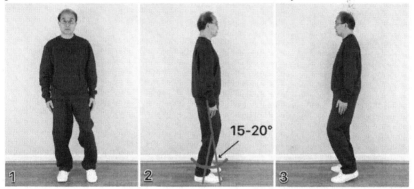

Figure 3-1C. Transitional Stance.

The Important Point. Bend your supporting knee to a lesser degree or do not flex it at all if you feel uncomfortable or pain in this stance.

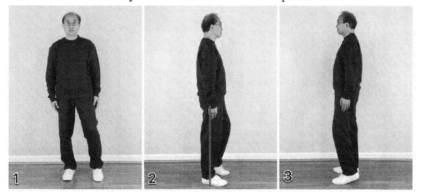

Figure 3-1Cc. Transitional Stance without rear knee flexion.

Stance Four: **Empty Stance**

Stand with the rear leg (the right leg in the figure) supporting the entire weight of the body. The rear knee is flexed at 10-20 degrees. The toes of the front foot (here the left foot) are placed in the front and pointed forward, and the rear foot (here the right foot) is angled outward at 35-45 degrees. See **Figure 3-1D**. It happens only in Posture Five. See Posture Five in Chapter 6.

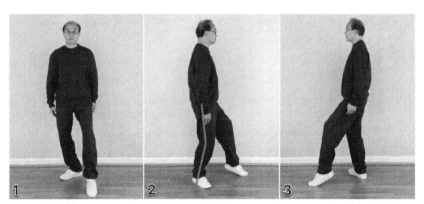

Figure 3-1D. Empty Stance.

The Important Point

Bend your rear knee to a lesser degree or do not flex it at all if you feel uncomfortable or pain in this stance.

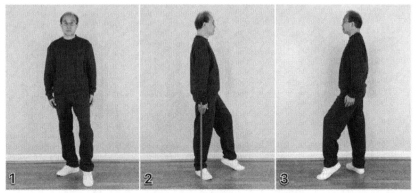

Figure 3-1Dd. Empty Stance without back knee flexion.

Stance Five: Bow Stance

If you walk forward slowly enough, you may find out that you adopt a bow stance that is seen in all styles of tai chi. Your front knee (the left knee in the figure) is mildly flexed with the front lower leg perpendicular to the ground and the back leg (here the right leg) straight. Your feet are shoulder-width apart with toes pointed forward. See **Figure 3-1E**. It is critical to perform this stance correctly. Otherwise, your knees will be damaged, as I mentioned before. See the explanations in the walking section.

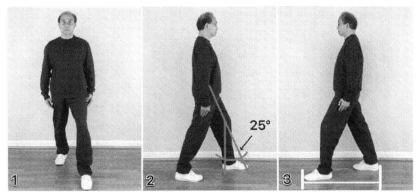

Figure 3-1E. Bow Stance.

The Important Point

Bend your front knee to a lesser degree and take shorter steps if you feel uncomfortable or pain in Bow Stance.

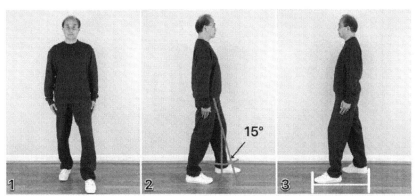

Figure 3-1Ee. Bow Stance with a lesser degree of knee flexion and a shorter step length.

83

Hands and Arms

Hands and Arms

Relax the hands with the fingers naturally positioned. See **Figure 3-2A**. Try to sink the shoulders and drop the elbows no matter what hand/arm movements you perform in tai chi. This is one of the most important tai chi principles, which helps not only relax your body and mind but make your postures look elegant. You will feel relaxed and energetic if you follow this simple rule. However, when doing stretching in Yoga E Tai Chi, you extend the fingers and arms fully. See **Figure 3-2Aa**.

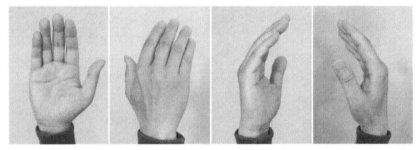

Figure 3-2A. Hands and fingers in E Tai Chi.

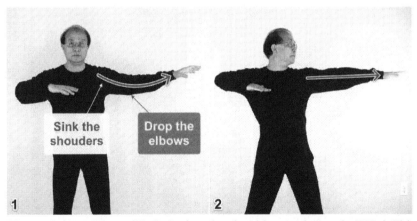

Figure 3-2Aa. **Photo #1**: Relaxing the shoulders and arms in E Tai Chi. **Photo #2**: Hands and arms during stretching in Yoga E Tai Chi.

Direction of palms

Whether your palms face downward, upward, outward, inward, or in any direction does not matter too much as long as you feel comfortable and relaxed. Different styles of tai chi prefer various directions of the palms. No scientific evidence has shown that palm-facing-upward is superior or palm-facing-downward is healthier.

In principle, your palms follow the direction of your hands. Your palm faces toward the front if you push your hand forward. Your palm faces upward when your hand is ascending. And your palm faces downward when your hand is descending. As you have become familiar with the hand/arm movements in E Tai Chi, your actions will direct your palms automatically and naturally without thinking. Of course, it is much easier to obtain "qi" when you follow this rule. I will demonstrate the direction of palm movements in Movement 1 and Movement 2, which give rise to all the other hand/arm movements in E Tai Chi.

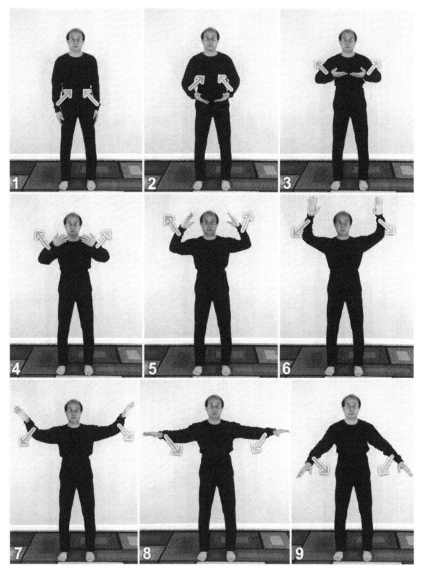

Figure 3-2B. Palm direction in Movement 1.

Key Points for **Figure 3-2B**.

Photo #1 to **Photo #3**. The palms face upward when the hands are ascending. **Photo #4**. Transition. The palms face backward. **Photo #5**. Transition. The palms face inward. **Photo #6**. Transition. The palms face forward. **Photo #7** to **Photo #9**. The palms face downward when the hands are descending.

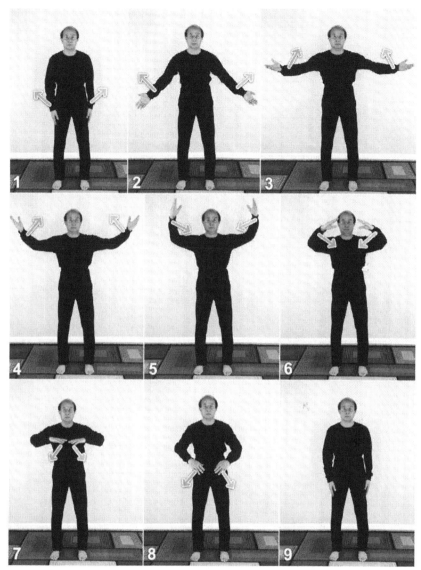

Figure 3-2C. Palm direction in Movement 2.

Key Points for **Figure 3-2C**.

Photo #1 to **Photo #3**. The palms face upward when the hands are ascending. **Photo #4**. Transition. The palms face inward. **Photo #5**. Transition. The palms face forward. **Photo #6** to **Photo #8**. The palms face downward when the hands are descending.

Hand and arm movements

They will be described in detail in Chapter 4.

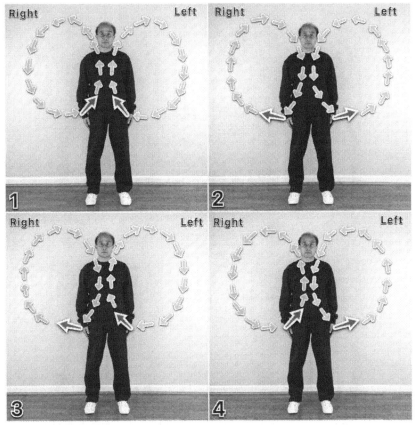

Figure 3-2D. Hand/Arm Movements 1, 2, and 3.

Photo #1. Movement 1. Simultaneously circle your left hand counterclockwise and right hand clockwise.

Photo #2. Movement 2. Simultaneously circle your left hand clockwise and right hand counterclockwise.

Photo #3. Movement 3 (Leftward). Simultaneously circle your left hand and right hand counterclockwise.

Photo #4. Movement 3 (Rightward). Simultaneously circle your left hand and right hand clockwise.

Walk

Walking is man's best medicine.

— Hippocrates (460–370 BC, Greek physician, father of modern medicine)

The typical traditional tai chi walk is a curved walk (see the diagram), which is hard to learn, not safe for older people, and has no health benefit. When you practice E Tai Chi, you can just walk naturally in any direction, slowly or fast.

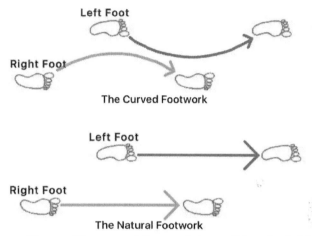

Upper Figure. The curved footwork in traditional tai chi.
Lower Figure. The footwork in natural walking and E Tai Chi.

Lift **the heel** up first and then the whole foot when you lift the foot to make a step. When performing slow walking in the E Tai Chi sequences, make sure not to over-flex the knee joint of the supporting front leg. This principle applies to any walking (forward, backward, and sideward).

Walking forward: Walk forward naturally with **the heel** hitting the ground first. See **Figure 3-3A**.

Walking backward: Walk backward naturally with **the toes** touching the ground first. See **Figure 3-3B**.

Walking sideways: Walk naturally to one side with **the toes** contacting the ground first, and then the whole foot. See **Figure 3-3C**.

Walking Forward

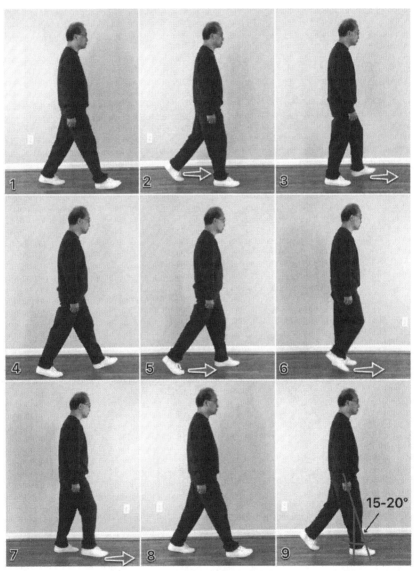

Figure 3-3A. Walking forward naturally.

Key points for **Figure 3-3A**.

Photo #1: **Initial Contact.** The right foot is moving forward with the right heel hitting the ground.

Photo #2: **Loading Response**. Shift the body weight to the right leg with the entire right foot contacting the ground. Lift the left heel up and get ready to step forward with the left foot.

Photo #3: **Midstance**. The left foot is swinging forward.

Photo #4: **Terminal Stance**. The left heel touches the ground. Gradually shift the body weight to the left leg.

Photo #5: **Preswing**. As the body weight has moved entirely to the left leg, the right heel comes off the ground. You are ready to step forward with the right foot.

Photo #6: **Initial Swing**. The right foot is swinging forward and passing the left foot.

Photo #7: **Midswing**. The right foot continues to move forward.

Photo #8 (= Photo #1): **Terminal Swing**. The right heel hits the ground. Now you can repeat the same cycle of normal forward-walking.

Photo #9: The same as **Photo #2 (Loading Response)**. The peak flexion of the knee.

Walking Backward

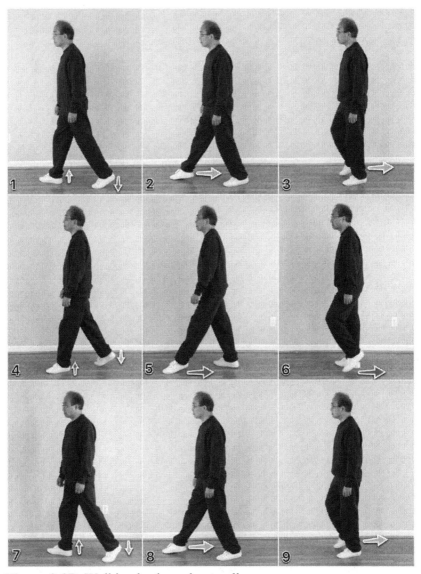

Figure 3-3B. Walking backward naturally.

Key points for **Figure 3-3B**.

Photo #1: The left foot is moving backward with the toes of the left foot touching the ground.

Photo #2: Shift the body weight to the left leg with the entire left foot contacting the ground. In the meantime, lift the right heel up and get ready to step back with the right foot.

(The left heel is naturally moved inward as the body weight is gradually shifted to the left leg. The inward movement of the heel should occur spontaneously because the resulting posture produces optimal body stability. The final posture is: the toes of the right foot, the front foot, are pointed forward, and the rear foot, the left foot, is angled outward at 35-45 degrees.)

Photo #3: The right foot is swinging backward. At this time, the right foot becomes parallel to the left foot.

Photo #4: The toes of the right foot touch the ground. Gradually shift the body weight to the right leg.

Photo #5: The body weight has moved entirely to the right leg. Lift the left heel up and get ready to step back with the left foot.

(The final posture is: the toes of the left foot (the front foot) are pointed forward, and the rear foot (the right foot) is angled outward at 35-45 degrees.)

Photo #6: The left foot is swinging backward and passing the right foot.

Photo #7(= Photo #1): The left foot continues to move backward and touches the ground with the toes of the left foot.

Photo #8 (= Photo #2): Shift your body weight to the left leg with the entire left foot contacting the ground. Lift the right heel up and get ready to step back with the right foot.

(The final posture is: the toes of the right foot (the front foot) are pointed forward, and the rear foot (the left foot) is angled outward at 35-45 degrees.)

Now you can repeat the same cycle of backward walking.

Photo #9= Photo #3.

Walking Sideways

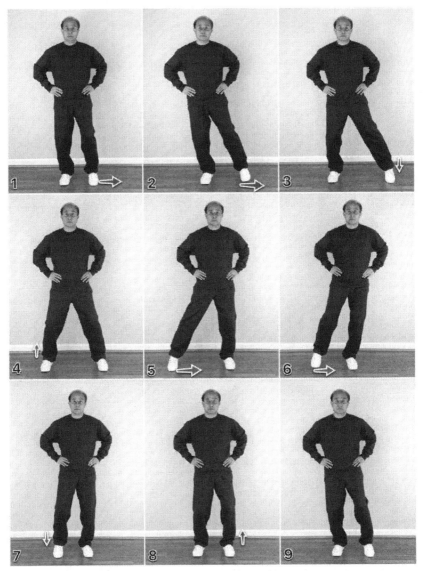

Figure 3-3C. Walking sideways (to the left).

Walk leftward. After you have shifted your weight to the right leg, take a step sideward left with your left foot. Lift the heel of the moving foot off the ground first and then the whole foot. The distance between your two feet is one to two feet wide. The toes of the left foot touch the

94

ground first, and then the whole foot contacts the ground. The toes of the feet keep facing forward.

After your left foot has become in complete contact with the ground, gradually shift your body weight to the left leg. Then, bring the right foot closer to the left foot and shift the weight back to the right leg. Repeat the same action if you continue to walk sideways left.

Walk rightward. Do it the same way with a different foot.

The above principle applies to all the sideward-moving postures (Postures One, Two, Three, Six, Seven, and Eight).

Key points for **Figure 3-3C**.

Photo #1: **Routine Stance** to **Transitional Stance**. Stand with feet shoulder-width apart. The knees are flexed at 10-20 degrees. Keep both feet pointed forward during walking sideways. Shift your body weight to the right leg. Lift the left heel up and get ready to step out.

Photo #2: Take a step sideways left with the left foot.

Photo #3: The toes of the left foot touch the ground.

Photo #4: Gradually shift the body weight to the left leg. At this moment, the weight is evenly distributed between both legs.

Photo #5: The body weight is completely shifted to the left leg with the right heel off the ground. You are ready to bring your right foot in.

Photo #6: Move the right foot toward the left foot.

Photo #7: The right foot comes in contact with the ground. The toes of the right foot touch the ground first. You are in **Transitional Stance** (the left leg is the supporting leg).

Photo #8: Gradually shift the body weight to the right leg. At this moment, the weight is evenly distributed between both legs. You are back to **Routine Stance**.

Photo #9: After having transferred your entire weight back to the right leg, you are in **Transitional Stance** again (the right leg is the supporting leg). You are ready to take the second sideward step with the left foot.

If you want to walk sideways to the right, then you can start by taking a step sideways right with the right foot in the same way as described above.

Slow Walking in E Tai Chi Sequences

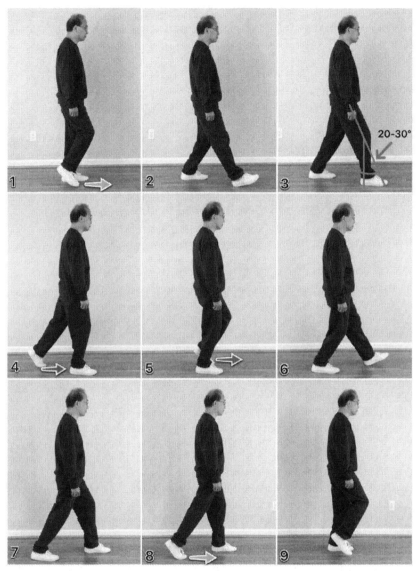

Figure 3-3D. Slow walking in E Tai Chi sequences.

Slow Walking in E Tai Chi Sequences

Keep the body upright. Lift **the heel** up first and then the whole foot when you lift the foot to make a step. This principle applies to any walking (forward, backward, and sideward).

Use the rear leg to push the body forward to shift the body weight to the front foot. This way will prevent the over-flexion of the supporting front leg. I propose that the flexion of the knees should not be over **20-30 degrees**, and the length of each step should be within **30 inches** (76 cm) in order to prevent knee injuries.

Key points for **Figure 3-3D**.

Photo #1: This is **Transitional Stance**: one of the legs (the left leg in the figure) is supporting the body weight while the toes of the other leg (here the right leg) gently touch the ground to maintain balance.

Photo #2: Step forward with the right foot. The right heel comes in contact with the ground.

Photo #3: Gradually shift the body weight to the right leg. Now, you are in **Bow Stance**: your front knee (here the right knee) is mildly flexed with the back leg (here the left leg) straight.

You should use the rear leg to push the body forward so that the front lower leg forms a 90-degree angle relative to the front foot or the ground. This is a standard **bow stance** in Chinese martial arts. When **you drive the body forward by the rear leg**, the front knee joint will not be over-flexed. This principle applies to all the forward movements.

Photo #4: As the body weight is fully shifted to the right leg, the left heel comes off the ground. You are ready to swing the left leg forward.

Photo #5: The left leg swings forward until it becomes parallel to the right leg. The toes of the left foot gently touch the ground. Now you are back in **Transitional Stance**.

Photo #6: Step forward with the left foot with the left heel hitting the ground.

Photo #7: Gradually shift the weight to the left leg. Again, you are in **Bow Stance**: your left knee (the front knee) is mildly flexed with the right leg (the back leg) straight.

Photo #8: As the body weight is fully shifted to the left leg, the right heel comes off the ground. You are ready to swing the right leg forward.

Photo #9: The right leg is swinging forward, and your right foot becomes parallel to the left foot (the front foot). The toes of the right foot (the back foot) gently touch the ground while the left foot continues to support the body. Now you are back in **Transitional Stance**.

Breathing

When feeling frustrated or overwhelmed, we would say, "Step back and take a deep breath." Definitely, slowing down our breathing helps calm your mind and reduce stress. The slow, deep, controlled breathing used in yoga and meditation has been shown to ease anxiety and depression. The lungs are the only internal organ we can control and manipulate voluntarily. A recent animal study indicates that the respiratory control center in the brain interacts with the other areas of the brain that are responsible for alertness and emotion (Yackle, et al., 2017). It provides scientific evidence for the effects of breathing exercises on our minds.

Traditional tai chi postures or yoga poses are not designed according to the rhythm of breath. Therefore, if emphasizing coordination of breath and movement when performing traditional tai chi postures or yoga poses, one has to carry out coordinated breathing and natural breathing alternately. The process is complicated to learn, and the breathing rhythms can be awkward. Since E Tai Chi or Yoga E Tai Chi consists of only symmetrical hand movements, you can synchronize your breathing with the hand movements from the beginning to the end easily and comfortably.

You should breathe spontaneously and naturally in the beginning. As you become familiar with the E Tai Chi or Yoga E Tai Chi movements, you can try to coordinate your hand movements with your breathing. In principle, breathe in when circling your arms up, and breathe out when circling your arms down. See **Figures 3-4A**. If you are performing alternate movements (Movement 4, 5, and 6), choose one of the arms as an indicator for breathing pattern, e.g., the left arm/hand.

When your arms are fully extended and stretched out, keep rotating your arms/shoulders. The arm rotating movements are perfectly coordinated with a breathing exercise. Inhale when rotating the arms to turn the palms upward and exhale when rotating the arms to turn the palms downward. See **Figures 3-4 B, C, and D**. Similarly, you exhale when turning the palms backward and inhale when turning the palms forward. See **Figure 3-4E**.

When coordinated with the hand movements in Yoga E Tai Chi, your breathing will be slow and deep if you practice them at the usual speed. A normal adult takes 12 to 16 breaths every minute at rest (Johns Hopkins Medicine, n.d.). For instance, the basic walking sequence of Yoga E Tai Chi consists of 40 movements. It usually takes approximately 8 to 10 minutes to finish the basic walking sequence. If you take 2 breaths when you perform each movement, then the total number of breaths you take during the execution of the sequence will be 80. Consequently, the respiration rate during Yoga E Tai Chi workouts will be 8 to 10 breaths per minute ($80/10 = 8$ or $80/8 = 10$). Surely, you can adjust the speed of the hand movements according to your conditions.

Numerous breathing methods have been described in yoga books. Almost all the yoga breathing methods are designed to be used in a sitting or lying position. Some of the yoga breathing techniques are challenging and dangerous. In order to make Yoga E Tai Chi as simple and safe as possible, I propose that you just breathe naturally, but at the same time, you consciously coordinate your breathing with your hand/arm movements. You do not need to think about which nostril is used or which muscles in the body are contracted in Yoga E Tai Chi.

The body energy, qi in tai chi, or prana in yoga was thought to travel or circulate through the energy centers (e.g., chakras) and channels (e.g., nadi). All these centers, channels, and qi/prana that are imagined by the ancient people haven't been proven scientifically. As the proverb says, "*All roads lead to Rome.*" You can imagine any route from the lower body to fingers or from fingers to the lower body. When you raise your hand or hands, you think that qi or prana moves starting from your lower body along the midline of the abdomen and chest, then it travels along the inner aspect of the shoulder, upper arm, elbow, forearm, wrist, palm, and finally, it reaches the tips of your fingers. When you drop your hands, qi/prana will travel along the same route but in the opposite direction: from fingers to the lower body.

I consider the sequential relaxing or stretching of your joints as the route of moving qi or prana, i.e., the route of a mindful exercise or meditation. Later on, you can practice the simple yoga breathing, **Three-Part Breath (dirgha pranayama)**:

Three-Part Breath. Breathe through your nose softly and slowly. Breathe into your belly, ribcage, and upper chest sequentially when you inhale. Namely, breathe in while expanding your abdomen, lower chest, and upper chest consecutively. When you exhale, reverse the above process: sequentially contract your upper chest, lower chest, and abdomen.

The process of breathing training can be summarized as follows:

Stage One: Breathe naturally;

Stage Two: Breathe naturally with coordination of hand movements.

Stage Three: Breathe naturally with coordination of hand movements and sequential relaxation or stretching of joints.

Stage Four: Practice Three-Part Breath with coordination of hand movements.

The above breathing exercises are natural, conscious, gentle, and effective because the slow and deep breathing is coordinated with the hand movements seamlessly. It is easy to learn, safe to practice, and comfortably applied to standing and walking Yoga E Tai Chi sequences. I am sure that you will achieve most of the health benefits of tai chi/yoga breathing by these simple breathing methods.

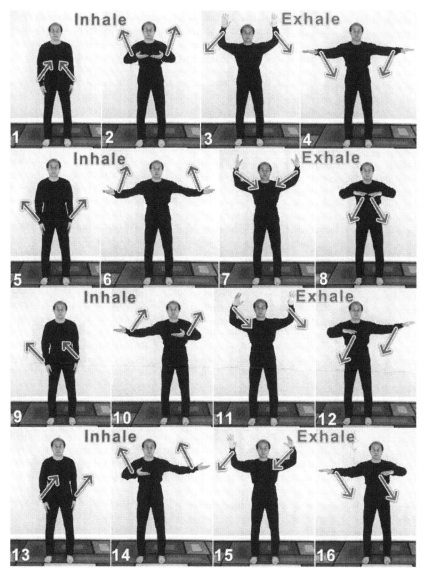

Figures 3-4A. Breathing coordinated with the circular hand movements.

Key Points for **Figure 3-4A**.

Photo#1 to **Photo#4**. Movement 1. Breathe in when the hands are going up. Breathe out when the hands are going down.

Photo#5 to **Photo#8**. Movement 2. Breathe in when the hands are going up. Breathe out when the hands are going down.

Photo#9 to **Photo #12**. Movement 3 (Leftward). Breathe in when the hands are going up. Breathe out when the hands are going down.

Photo#13 to **Photo#16**. Movement 3 (Rightward). Breathe in when the hands are going up. Breathe out when the hands are going down.

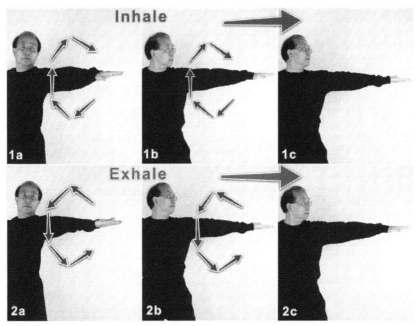

Figures 3-4B. Breathing coordinated with the arm rotations in Sideward Movement 1.

Key Points for **Figure 3-4B**.

Photos #1a (Oblique View) and **#1b**: The palms are facing downward. Inhale while rotating the arms to turn the palms upward (supinating).

Photo #1c: The palms have been turned to face upward.

Photos #2a (Oblique View) and **#2b**: The palms are facing upward. Exhale while rotating the arms to turn the palms downward (pronating).

Photo #2c: The palms have been turned to face downward.

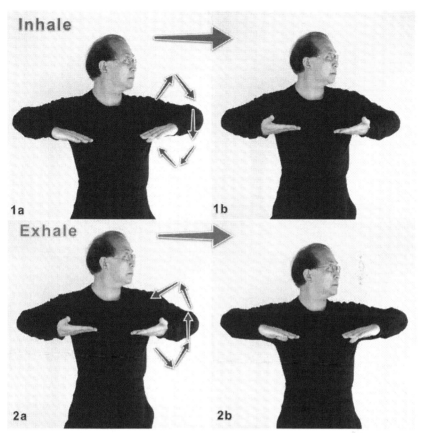

Figure Figures 3-4C. Breathing coordinated with the arm rotations in Sideward Movement 2.

Key Points for **Figure 3-4C**.

Photo #1a: The palms are facing downward. Inhale while rotating the arms to turn the palms upward (supinating).

Photo #1b: The palms have been turned to face upward.

Photo #2a: The palms are facing upward. Exhale while rotating the arms to turn the palms downward (pronating).

Photo #2b: The palms have been turned to face downward.

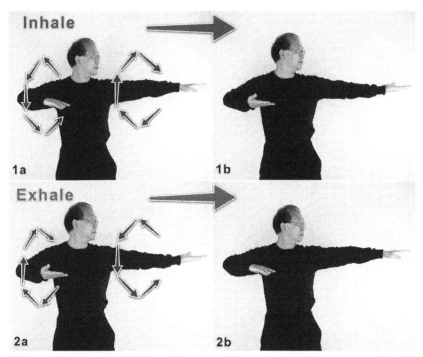

Figure Figures 3-4D Breathing coordinated with the arm rotations in Sideward Movement 3.

Key Points for **Figure 3-4D**.

Photo #1a: The palms are facing downward. Inhale while rotating the arms to turn the palms upward (supinating).

Photo #1b: The palms have been turned to face upward.

Photo #2a: The palms are facing upward. Exhale while rotating the arms to turn the palms downward (pronating).

Photo #2b: The palms have been turned to face downward.

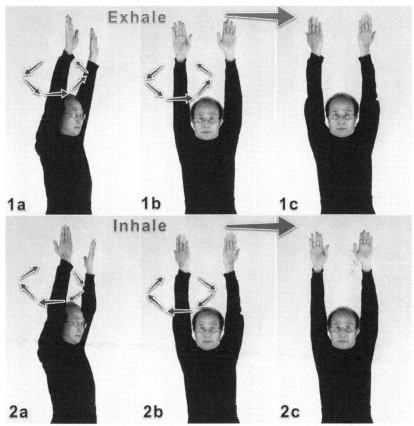

Figures 3-4E. Breathing coordinated with the arm rotations in Upward Movement 1 and Backward Movement 2.

Key Points for **Figure 3-4E**.

Photos #1a (Oblique View) and **#1b**: The palms are facing forward. Exhale while rotating the arms to turn the palms backward (supinating).

Photo #1c: The palms have been turned to face backward.

Photos #2a (Oblique View) and **#2b**: The palms are facing backward. Inhale while rotating the arms to turn the palms forward (pronating).

Photo #2c: The palms have been turned to face forward.

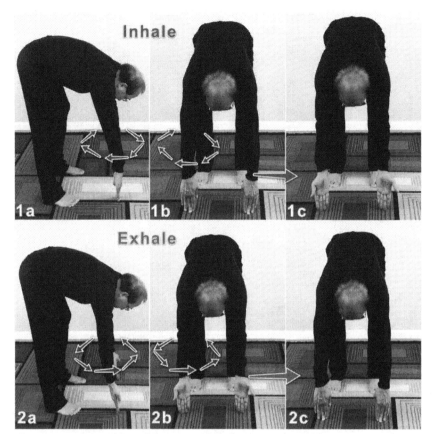

Figure 3-4F. Breathing coordinated with the arm rotations in Downward Movement 2.

Key Points for **Figure 3-4F**.

Photos #1a (Lateral View) and **#1b**: The palms are facing backward. Inhale while rotating the arms to turn the palms forward (supinating).

Photo #1c: The palms have been turned to face forward.

Photos #2a (Lateral View) and **#2b**: The palms are facing forward. Exhale while rotating the arms to turn the palms backward (pronating).

Photo #1c: The palms have been turned to face backward.

Chapter 4. Hand/Arm Movements
(also Used in Yoga E Tai Chi)

早发白帝城
朝辞白帝彩云间，千里江陵一日还。
两岸猿声啼不住，轻舟已过万重山。

LEAVING THE WHITE KING'S TOWN AT DAWN

Leaving at dawn the White King crowned with rainbow cloud,
I have sailed a thousand miles through Three Georges in a day.
With monkeys' sad adieus the riverbanks are loud;
My boat has left ten thousand mountains far away.

—李白 (Li Bai, 701－762, Chinese poet)
Translated by 许渊冲 (Xu Yuanchong)

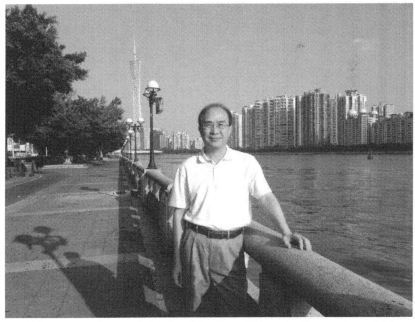

Walking along the north bank of the Pearl River in Guangzhou, China.

All the tai chi movements can be condensed to one circular hand movement. Thus, E Tai Chi requires only **one** basic hand movement: circle your hands in front of your body. However, you will have a total of six different hand movements when you circle your hands simultaneously, sequentially, clockwise, or counterclockwise.

In this book, I circle my left hand and right hand on the left and right sides of my body, respectively, in order to clearly demonstrate the six hand movements and facilitate the learning process. However, when you perform the circular hand/arm movements, your hands or arms can be overlapped (crossed over the midline of your body) as long as you feel good. What you feel comfortable is right. Again, there is no strict rule in E Tai Chi. E Tai Chi is for your personal health only, not for fighting or competition. As a matter of fact, these six hand movements include all the fighting techniques in traditional tai chi.

Usually, you perform these circular hand movements vertically in front of your body because most of the typical tai chi hand movements are performed this way. Therefore, I focus on demonstrating the vertical hand movements. However, you can play them diagonally, horizontally, or in any direction you like. In the advanced E Tai Chi, you perform the hand movements both vertically and horizontally. You will be surprised that tai chi can be practiced this way or any way you want.

As mentioned previously, whether your palms face downward, upward, outward, inward, or in any direction does not matter too much if you feel comfortable and relaxed. Different styles of tai chi prefer various directions of the palms. No scientific evidence shows that palm-facing-up is superior, or the palm-facing-down is healthier.

In principle, your palms follow the direction of your hands. Your palm faces toward the front if you push your hand forward. The palm faces upward when the hand is ascending. And the palm faces downward when the hand is descending. It is much easier to obtain "qi" when you follow this rule. The concept of "qi" (energy?) will be discussed in the science book.

The distance between your face/chest and your hands is usually about 1 foot (30 cm). However, you can use any range you want.

There are only six hand movements in E Tai Chi. It's simple, right? One of these movements (Movement 4) is **Cloud Hands (Wave Hands like Clouds)**, which exists in all styles of tai chi and is executed in a similar way: sequentially circle your hands up in front of your torso. Principally, all the tai chi movements should look like floating clouds if you can perform them well. I would call Movement 4 "**Standard Cloud Hands**."

Nowadays, "cloud" is a hot name. We have cloud computing, cloud storage, and cloud-based anything. Hence, I call the remaining five movements "Cloud Hands" too, but with some modifiers. I can guarantee that these five movements are completely brand new, and no one has practiced them this way before. For example, all tai chi practitioners move their hands vertically to perform Standard Cloud Hands. Why can't we circle our hands horizontally, obliquely, or in the reverse direction? What tai chi masters did or what tai chi teachers taught is not the only way one can practice tai chi well and creatively. This is the reason that there are so many tai chi styles.

However, only in E Tai Chi, you can practice tai chi creatively. **The rule is "no rule" in E Tai Chi.** After you have learned the basics, you can practice E Tai Chi any way you desire. You can design E Tai Chi sequences by yourself. No one will say that you are performing E Tai Chi the wrong way. Again, E Tai Chi means simple, safe, and gentle.

If you **simultaneously** circle your hands up through the midline of the body (the left-hand circles counterclockwise and the right hand clockwise), you are doing **Movement 1**, which I call "**Ascending Cloud Hands**." See **Photo #1** in **Figure 4-0A**.

If you **simultaneously** circle your hands up to your sides (the right-hand circles counterclockwise and the left hand clockwise), you are doing **Movement 2**, which I call "**Descending Cloud Hands**." See **Photo #2** in **Figure 4-0A**.

When you **simultaneously** circle your hands to the left or the right (both hands circle counterclockwise or clockwise), you are performing **Movement 3,** which I name "**Concurrent Cloud Hands**." See **Photo #3** and **Photo#4** in **Figure 4-0A**.

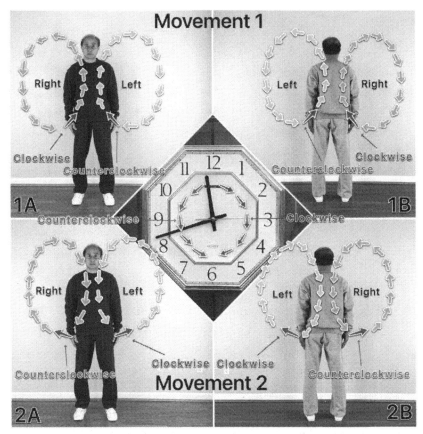

Figure 4-00. Clarification of the hand motions in E Tai Chi. The arrows show the direction of hand movements. The large arrows indicate the starting points of hand movements. All the hand/arm movements in E Tai Chi are based on Movement 1 and Movement 2.

Photos 1A (front view) and **1B** (back view). **Movement 1**: simultaneously circle your hands up through the midline of the body and circle your hands down and out to your sides (simultaneously circle your left hand **counterclockwise** and your right hand **clockwise**).

Photos 2A (front view) and **2B** (back view). **Movement 2**: simultaneously circle your hands up, out to your sides, and circle your hands down along the midline of the body (simultaneously circle your left hand **clockwise** and your right hand **counterclockwise**).

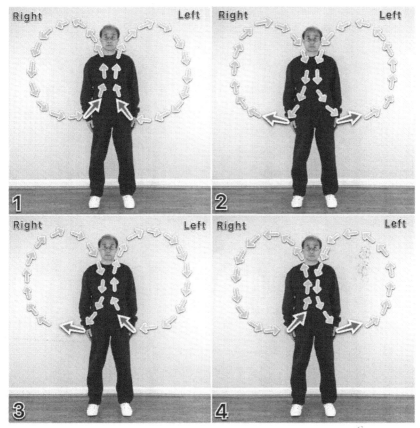

Figure 4-0A. The motions of Movements 1, 2, and 3. The arrows show the direction of hand movements. The large arrows indicate the starting points of hand movements.

Photo #1. Movement 1: simultaneously circle your hands up through the midline of the body and circle your hands down and out to your sides (simultaneously circle your left hand counterclockwise and your right hand clockwise).

Photo #2. Movement 2: simultaneously circle your hands up, out to your sides, and circle your hands down along the midline of the body (simultaneously circle your left hand clockwise and your right hand counterclockwise).

Photos #3 and **#4. Movement 3**: simultaneously circle your hands in the same direction (counterclockwise or clockwise) in front of the body.

If you **sequentially** circle your hands up in front of your torso (left-hand circles counterclockwise and right-hand clockwise), you will get Movement 4, which is traditionally called "**Wave Hands like Clouds, or Cloud Hands**." See **Photo #1** in **Figure 4-0B**.

If you **sequentially** circle up your hands to the sides of your body (right-hand circles counterclockwise and left-hand clockwise), you will get **Movement 5**, which I name "**Reverse Cloud Hands**." See **Photo #2** in **Figure 4-0B**

If you **sequentially** circle up one hand in front of the torso and another hand to the side, then you will have **Movement 6**, which I call "**Bidirectional Cloud Hands**." See **Photos #3-#4** in **Figure 4-0B**.

The six E Tai Chi hand movements are summarized as follows:
Movement 1: Ascending Cloud Hands,
Movement 2: Descending Cloud Hands,
Movement 3: Concurrent Cloud Hands,
Movement 4: Standard Cloud Hands,
Movement 5: Reverse Cloud Hands,
Movement 6: Bidirectional Cloud Hands.

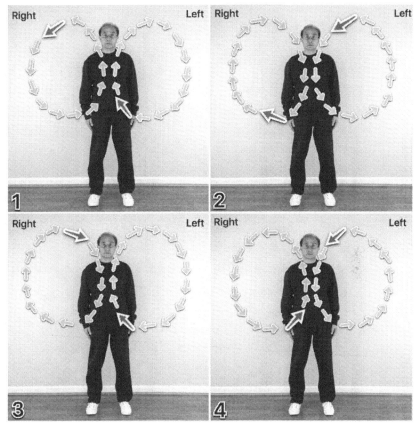

Figure 4-0B. The motions of Movements 4, 5, and 6. The arrows show the direction of hand movements. The large arrows indicate the starting points of hand movements.

Key Points for **Figure 4-0B**

Photo #1. Movement 4: sequentially circle your hands up through the midline of the body (sequentially circle your left hand counterclockwise and your right hand clockwise).

Photo #2. Movement 5: sequentially circle your hands up, out to your sides (sequentially circle your left hand clockwise and your right hand counterclockwise).

Photo #3. Leftward Movement 6: sequentially circle your hands in the same direction (counterclockwise) in front of the body.

Photo #4. Rightward Movement 6: sequentially circle your hands in the same direction (clockwise) in front of the body.

Now you have known these six hand movements in E Tai Chi. That's it! However, I will explain how to perform them in detail later.

Movements 1, 2, and 3 are so simple that you can learn how to do them within minutes. If you do not want to go further, you can practice standing or walking E Tai Chi right away. That means you perform Movements 1, 2, and 3 while standing or walking naturally.

Furthermore, you can master the basic E Tai Chi sequence within an hour. You can tell your friends and family members that you know how to practice tai chi and enjoy it.

Because you can learn and enjoy E Tai Chi with minutes or hours, you will have the confidence to continue to learn more and avoid the failure many tai chi learners have suffered due to the awkward beginning movements in all the tai chi styles.

If you can practice the standing or walking E Tai Chi, and the basic E Tai Chi sequence every day for 20-30 minutes, you will achieve almost all the health benefits of tai chi.

Certainly, performing the somewhat complicated movements like Movements 4, 5, and 6 will build up your confidence and make you enjoy more the beauty of tai chi. Even though Movements 4, 5, and 6 appear difficult, you can learn them within 1-2 hours. The fluidity of the movements, the relaxation of the body, and coordination of leg/arm movements can be gradually mastered as you practice E Tai Chi regularly.

Here, you will learn how to practice the standard Movements 1 to 3 used in E Tai Chi. After you have learned these standard movements, it is very straightforward for you to practice in a **yoga-tai chi** way. When you study the standing and walking postures in Chapters 5 and 6, I will show you step by step how to integrate the yoga components into the above hand movements.

The instructions for Movements 4, 5, and 6 will be found in the advanced book of Yoga E Tai Chi.

Movement 1: Ascending Cloud Hands

Let us start to practice it. Simultaneously raise both hands up in front of your torso slowly and comfortably. Your hands move upward in a circular manner toward the midline. After your hands meet at upper abdomen or chest level, spread your hands out and raise them overhead or to any height you like. Then, move your hands circularly downward and outward, and gently drop them back to your sides.

In other words, simultaneously circle your right hand clockwise and your left hand circles counterclockwise in front of your body. It does not matter how close or far your hands/arms are away from your body if you feel comfortable. Similarly, you do not need to worry about how high your hands will ascend although the most natural and comfortable height of your hands is at the level of your head or slightly overhead.

In principle, your palms follow the direction of your hands. Your palm faces toward the front if you push your hand forward. The palm faces upward when the hand is ascending, and it faces downward when the hand is descending. The distance between your face/chest and your hands is usually about 1 foot (30 cm). You are done with the first movement, Movement 1.

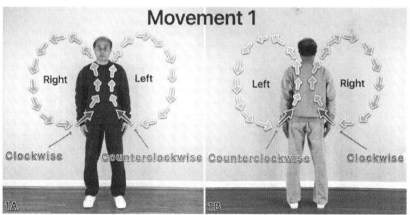

Photo 1A and **1B**. Movement 1: simultaneously circle your left hand counterclockwise and your right hand clockwise. The large red arrows indicate the starting points of hand movements.

115

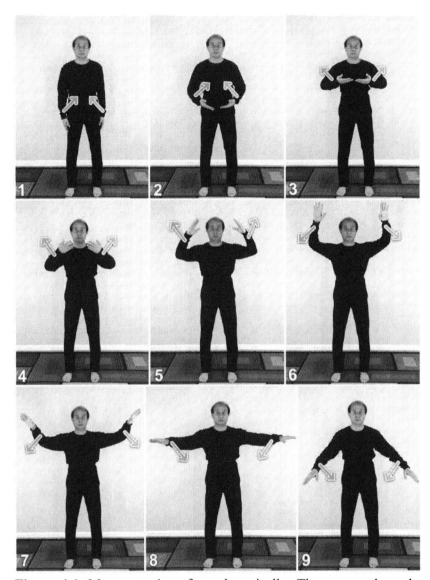

Figure 4-1. Movement 1 performed vertically. The arrows show the direction of hand movements.

Key points for **Figure 4-1**.

Photo #1: Normal Standing. Stand with feet shoulder-width apart. Your hands rest at your sides. The knees are straight. Keep your torso upright. This is the starting stance for the following actions.

Photo #2: Circle your hands up through the midline of your body. The palms are directed upward when the hands are ascending. The fingers of both hands point to each other diagonally. You look like you are holding a big ball in front of your body.

Photo #3: The hands continue to ascend. They are at shoulder level at this moment.

Photo #4: When your hands are raised above the chest, your palms gradually turn (pronate) and face backward.

Photo #5: The palms are directed to face inwards during the transition from facing upward to facing forward.

Photo #6: When the hands are lifted above the head, the palms turn to face forward. You look like you are pushing the ball away.

Photo #7: The palms face downward while the hands are descending to your sides. However, you do not have to think about the direction of the palms at all in the beginning. Do whatever you feel comfortable.

Photo #8: The hands continue to descend. They are at shoulder level at this moment.

Photo #9: The hands are returning to your sides.

Movement 2: Descending Cloud Hands

This movement is almost the same as Movement 1 except moving in the opposite direction.

Simultaneously spread and raise your arms to the sides in a circular manner outwardly and upwardly. At chest level, your hands move circularly up and toward the midline until they are lifted above the head. Then, your hands start to go inward and downward in front of the torso. Finally, your hands gently drop back to your sides.

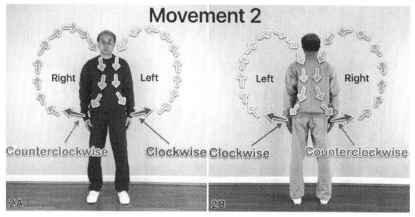

Photos 2A and **2B**. Movement 2: simultaneously circle your left hand clockwise and your right hand counterclockwise. The large red arrows indicate the starting points of hand movements.

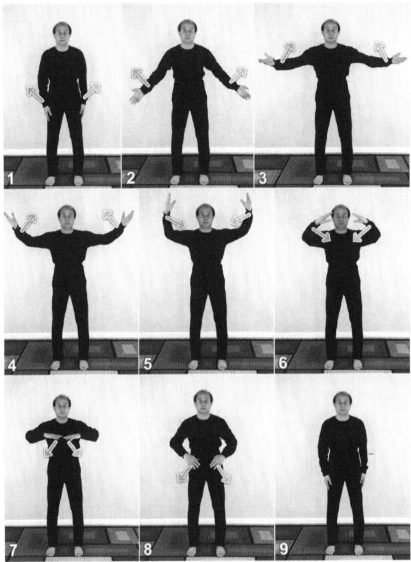

Figure 4-2. Movement 2 performed vertically. The arrows show the direction of hand movements.

Key points for **Figure 4-2**

Photo #1: **Normal Standing**. Stand naturally with feet shoulder-width apart.

Photo #2: Your hands are circling up to the sides. As the arms rotate out, the palms gradually turn and face forward.

Photo #3: The hands continue to ascend with the palms facing upward. The hands are at shoulder level at this moment.

Photo #4: The palms face inward as the hands are raised above shoulder level.

Photo #5: When the hands are raised overhead, the palms turn to face forward. Hereafter, the hands start to descend through the midline of the body.

Photo #6: The hands continue to incline through the midline with the palms facing downward.

Photo #7: The hands are at shoulder level.

Photo #8: The hands are returning to your sides.

Photo #9: Your hands have returned to your sides. You are back to **Normal Standing**.

Movement 3: Concurrent Cloud Hands

Circle both arms vertically in front of your body continuously. In other words, both hands move together in the same direction, clockwise or counterclockwise.

If your hands move circularly toward the left, then you realized you are practicing Movement 1 with your left arm and Movement 2 with your right arm. Similarly, if your hands move circularly toward the right, then you are practicing Movement 1 with your right arm and Movement 2 with your left arm. Namely, simultaneously practicing Movement 1 and Movement 2 with different hands is equal to practicing Movement 3.

Movement 1 + Movement 2 = Movement 3.

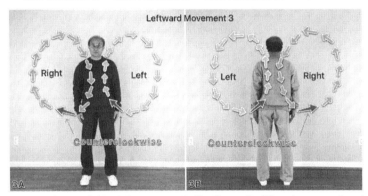

Photos 3A and **3B**. Movement 3 (Leftward): Simultaneously circle your left hand and right hand counterclockwise.

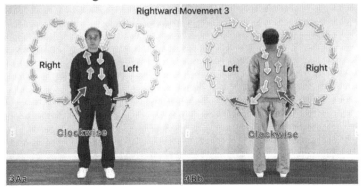

Photos 3Aa and **3Bb**. Movement 3 (Rightward): Simultaneously circle your left hand and right hand clockwise.

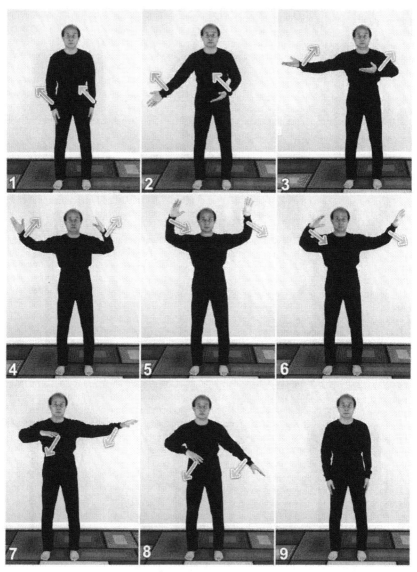

Figure 4-3A. Leftward Movement 3 performed vertically. The arrows show the direction of hand movements.

Key points for **Figure 4-3A**

Leftward Movement 3. Both hands simultaneously circle counterclockwise in front of the body.

Photo #1: **Normal Standing**. Stand naturally with feet shoulder-width apart.

Photo #2: Your right hand circles up to the side while your left hand circles up through the midline of the body.

Photo #3: The hands continue to ascend with the palms facing upward.

Photo #4: The palms face inward as the hands raised above shoulder level.

Photo #5: The hands have raised above the head with the palms facing forward. Hereafter, the right hand starts to descend through the midline while the left hand moves down to the side.

Photo #6: The hands continue to incline with the palms facing downward.

Photo #7: The hands are at shoulder level.

Photo #8: The hands are returning to your sides.

Photo #9: Your hands have returned to your sides. You are back to **Normal Standing**.

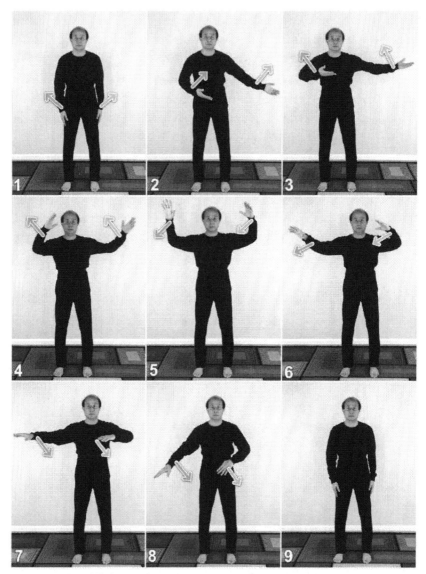

Figure 4-3B. Rightward Movement 3 performed vertically. The arrows show the direction of hand movements.

Chapter 5. Standing Postures in Yoga E Tai Chi

Worry only about the things that are in your control, the things that can be influenced and changed by your actions, not about the things that are beyond your capacity to direct or alter.

—M. A. Soupios and Panos Mourdoukoutas
(Authors of *The Ten Golden Rules: Ancient Wisdom from the Greek Philosophers on Living the Good Life*) (Mourdoukoutas, 2012)

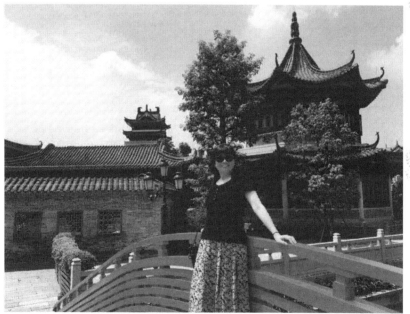

Visiting the Cantonese Opera Art Museum in Guangzhou, China.

As mentioned before, you can practice Yoga E Tai Chi anywhere, in the park, in the office, in the backyard, in the living room, and even in the bathroom.

All the standing postures are started in **Routine Stance**. Stand naturally in a relaxed state with your feet shoulder-width apart. Your hands and arms hang loosely at your sides. Gently bend your knees at a 10-20-degree angle. Keep your eyes looking straight ahead and breathe naturally and peacefully. Then, you are ready to practice the standing Yoga E Tai Chi postures.

Actually, you can practice the standing postures in a seated position if space is limited (e.g., in the office) or if you have any medical condition that does not allow you to stand up. How long you hold a pose is up to you. Bend your knees to a lesser degree or do not flex your knees at all if you feel uncomfortable or pain in Routine Stance or Transitional Stance. Try to do the stretching exercises according to your flexibility and comfort.

You do not need to think about the direction of palms and breathing coordination at all in the beginning. Do whatever you feel comfortable.

Here, I introduce eight standing postures, which are derived from the corresponding yoga poses.

Upward Movement1 is derived from Raised Hands Pose (Urdhva Hastasana);

Forward Movement 1 from Warrior 1 Pose (Virabhadrasana I);

Sideward Movement 1 from Warrior 2 Pose (Virabhadrasana II);

Sideward Movement 2 from Mountain Pose (Tadasana) variations;

Sideward Movement 3 from Archer Pose;

Backward Movement 2 from Raised Arms Pose (Hasta Uttanasana);

Downward Movement 2 from Standing Forward Bend (Uttanasana);

Balance Postures from Tree Pose (Vriksasana) or its variations.

You can perform all the standing postures one by one. Or you may select some of the postures and practice them in a sequence. Namely, you can sequence the standing postures anyway you like.

For example, Upward Movement 1→Forward Movement 1→

Sideward Movement 1→Backward Movement 2→

Balance Movement 2→Downward Movement 2.

I will provide step-by-step instructions for every Yoga E Tai Chi posture. However, I give only a brief description of each yoga pose adopted here. You should refer to other standard yoga books if you want to know how to perform the regular yoga poses mentioned in this book.

Upward and Forward Postures

Standing Upward Movement 1

The yoga component of this posture is derived from **Raised Hands Pose** (Urdhva Hastasana). Please review **Movement 1**: simultaneously circle your hands up through the midline of the body and circle your hands down and out to your sides. See the details in Chapter 4.

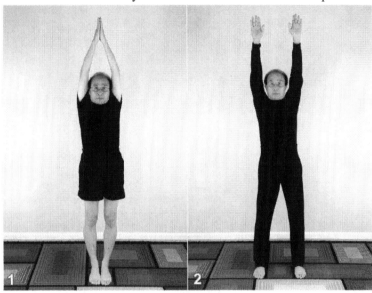

Figure 5-1A. **Photo #1**: **Raised Hands Pose** (Urdhva Hastasana). Stand with your big toes touching and your heels slightly apart. Raise your hands overhead with your elbows fully extended and your palms pressed together.

Photo #2: The yoga component of **Upward Movement 1**. Stand with your feet shoulder-width apart and your knees straight. Raise your hands overhead with your elbows fully extended and your palms facing forward. Keep your eyes looking forward or upward. See the following detailed instructions on how to perform Upward Movement 1.

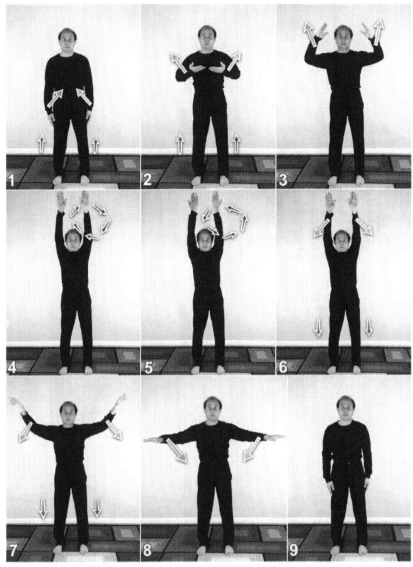

Figure 5-1B. Standing Upward Movement 1 (front view).

Key points for **Figure 5-1B** and **Figure 5-1C**.

Photo #1: Routine Stance. Stand with feet shoulder-width apart. Your hands rest at your sides. The knees are flexed at 10-20 degrees. Keep your torso upright.

Photos #2: Slowly straighten your knee joints when you are raising your hands through the midline (**Movement 1**). The palms are directed upward when the hands are ascending. The fingers of both hands point to each other diagonally. You look like you are holding a big ball in front of your body. **Inhale** while raising the hands.

Photo #3: When your hands are raised above shoulder level, your palms gradually turn (pronate) to face inward during the transition from facing upward to facing forward.

Photo #4: As your hands are raised overhead and fully extended, the palms are directed forwards, and the knees are straight. Keep your eyes looking forward or upward.

If you have strong legs, stand on tiptoe while holding this pose. This pose looks like **Raised Hands Pose** in yoga and many postures in qigong. Hold this pose for one breath or as many breaths as you like.

Hereafter, **exhale** and slowly rotate your arms to turn the palms backward (supinate) while keeping your arms straightened. You do not need to think about breathing coordination in the beginning. Just breathe spontaneously.

Photo #5: Your palms have been turned to face backward. Next, **inhale** and rotate your arms to turn the palms forward (pronate) again.

Photo #6: Your palms have been turned to face forward. From now, **exhale** and lower your arms to the sides while turning the palms downward (pronate).

Photo #7: You are dropping your hands with the palms facing downward. At the same time, gradually bend your knee joints and exhale slowly.

Photo #8: The hands continue to descend with the palms facing downward. The hands are at shoulder level at this moment.

Photo #9: The hands have returned to your sides with the knees gently flexed. You are back to **Routine Stance** and ready to perform the next posture.

Breathing Coordination.

Photos #1, **#2**, and **#3**: Inhale while raising the hands.

Photo #4: Exhale while turning the palms backward (supinate).

Photo #5: Inhale while turning the palms forward (pronate).

Photos #6, **#7**, and **#8**: Exhale while lowering the hands.

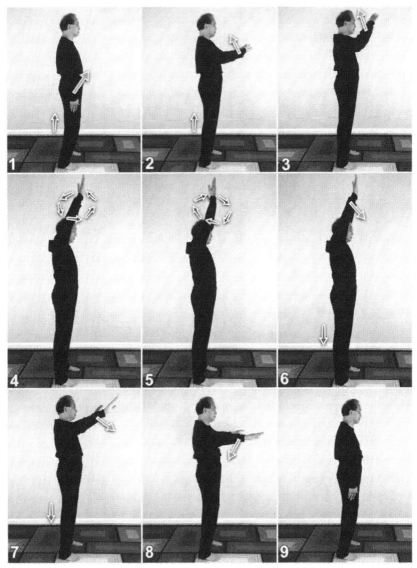

Figure 5-1C. Standing Upward Movement 1 (lateral view)

The Important Point

Bend your knees to a lesser degree or do not flex them at all if you feel uncomfortable or pain in Routine Stance. Raise your hands to any height that is comfortable for you if you have shoulder pain or injury.

Standing Forward Movement 1

The yoga component of this posture is derived from **Warrior 1 Pose** (Virabhadrasana I). Please review **Movement 1**: simultaneously circle your hands up through the midline of the body and circle your hands down and out to your sides. See the details in Chapter 4.

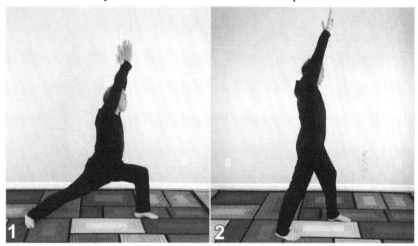

Figure 5-1D.

Photo #1: **Warrior 1 Pose** (Virabhadrasana I). Extend your arms upward with the palms facing each other or pressed together. Bend your front knee 90 degrees and straighten your back leg. The front knee is directly over the front ankle. The rear foot is turned in approximately 60-90 degrees, and the tip of the front foot is pointed forward. The heel of the front foot is aligned with the heel or the arch of the back foot. Gaze forward or up toward your hands.

Photo #2: The yoga component of **Forward Movement 1**. Raise your arms over the head with the palms facing forward. The elbows are fully extended. Gently flex your front knee with the front lower leg perpendicular to the ground and the back leg straight. Your feet are shoulder-width apart with the tips of your feet pointed forward. Gaze forward.

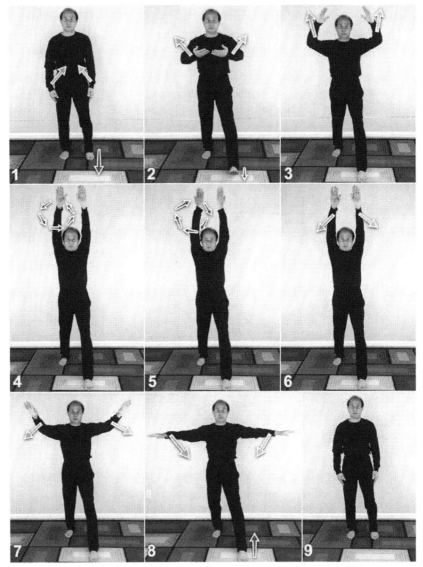

Figure 5-1E. Standing Forward Movement 1(front view). Step forward with the left foot.

Key points for **Figure 5-1E** and **Figure 5-1F**.

Photo #1: Normal Standing. Stand with feet shoulder-width apart. Your hands rest at your sides. Shift your weight to the right leg and be in **Transitional Stance** and get ready to step forward with the left foot.

Photo #2: Take a step forward with your left foot while circling your hands up through the midline (**Movement 1**). **Inhale** while raising the hands. Your left heel is hitting the ground, and the hands are at shoulder level.

Photo #3: When your hands are raised above shoulder level, your palms gradually turn (pronate) to face inward. Gradually shift your weight to the left leg.

Photo #4: As your left foot comes in complete contact with the ground, shift your weight to the left leg. When shifting the body weight from the right leg to the left leg, you should use the rear leg (here the right leg) to push the body forward so that the front lower leg (here the left leg) forms a 90-degree angle relative to the ground. This is a typical **bow stance** in Chinese martial arts. When **you drive the body forward by the rear leg**, the front knee joint will not be over-flexed.

At this time, your hands are raised overhead and fully extended with the palms facing forward. Keep your eyes looking forward or upward. This pose looks like **Warrior 1 Pose** in yoga. Hold this pose for one breath or as many breaths as you like.

Hereafter, **exhale** and slowly rotate your arms to turn the palms backward (supinate) while keeping your arms straightened.

Photo #5: Your palms have been turned to face backward. Next, **inhale** while rotating your arms to turn the palms forward (pronate) again.

Photo #6: Your palms have been turned to face forward. Then, **exhale** and lower your arms with the palms facing downward. Gradually shift your weight back to the right leg while dropping your hands.

Photo #7: Your hands are descending to the sides, and your weight is shifting to the right leg (the rear leg).

Photo #8: The hands have lowered to shoulder level with the palms facing downward. As your body weight has been completely shifted to the right leg, the left heel comes off the ground. You are ready to withdraw your left foot.

Photo #9: Your left foot has moved back and become parallel to the right foot. Your hands have returned to your sides with the knees gently flexed. At this moment, the body weight is evenly distributed between your legs. You are back to **Routine Stance** and ready to perform the next posture.

Breathing Coordination. Photos #1, **#2**, and **#3**: Inhale while raising the hands. **Photo #4**: Exhale while turning the palms backward (supinate). **Photo #5**: Inhale while turning the palms forward (pronate). **Photos #6**, **#7**, and **#8**: Exhale while dropping the hands.

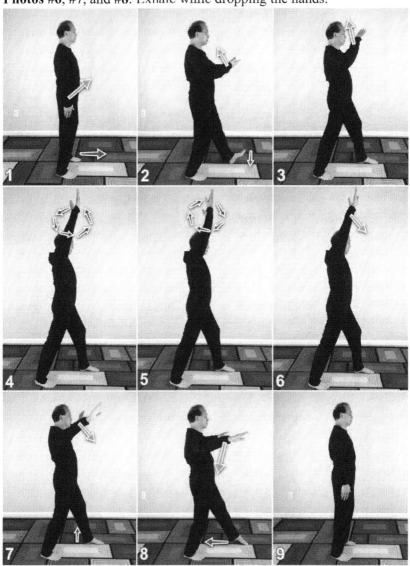

Figure 5-1F. Standing Forward Movement 1 (lateral view). Step forward with the left foot.

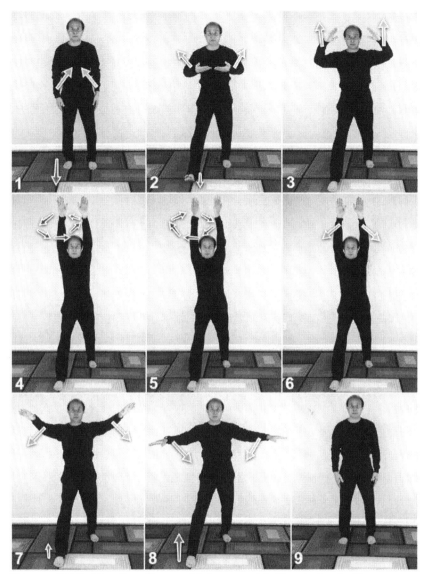

Figure 5-1G. Standing Forward Movement 1 (front view). Step forward with the **right foot**.

The Important Point

Bend your front knee to a lesser degree and take shorter steps if you feel uncomfortable or pain in **Bow Stance**. Raise your hands to any height that is comfortable for you if you have shoulder pain or injury.

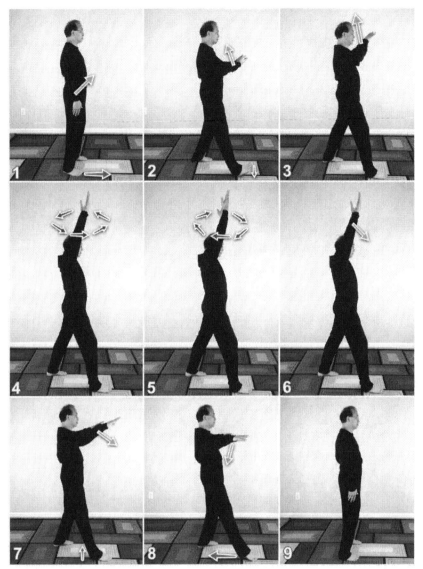

Figure 5-1H. Standing Forward Movement 1 (lateral view). Step forward with the **right foot**.

Sideward Postures

Standing Sideward Movement 1

The yoga component of this posture is derived from **Warrior 2 Pose** (Virabhadrasana II). Please review the execution of **Movement 1** in Chapter 4.

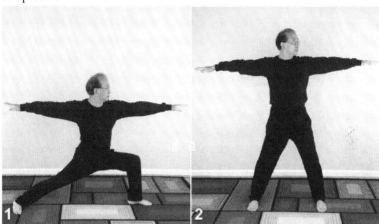

Figure 5-2A. **Photo #1**: **Warrior 2 Pose** (Virabhadrasana II). Extend your arms out to the sides and make them parallel to the ground with your palms facing down. Bend your front knee 90 degrees and straighten your back leg. The front knee is directly over the front ankle. The rear foot is turned in approximately 60-90 degrees, and the tip of the front foot is pointed leftward. The heel of the front foot is aligned with the heel or the arch of the back foot. Gaze over the middle finger of your front hand.

Photo #2: The yoga component of **Sideward Movement 1**. Stand with your feet one to two feet apart and pointed forward. The front knee (the left knee in the figure) is mildly bent, and the back knee is straight. Both feet are in complete contact with the floor. Spread your arms in a straight line at shoulder level. Your arms are parallel to the floor with the palms facing downward. Keep your eyes looking over the mid-finger of the front hand.

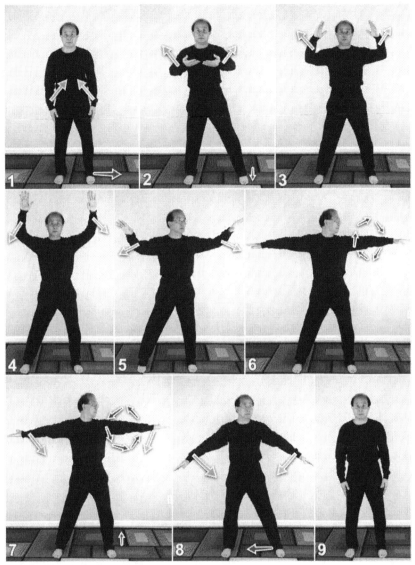

Figure 5-2B. Standing Sideward Movement 1. Take a side step with the left foot while performing Movement 1.

Key points for **Figure 5-2B.**

Photo #1: **Routine Stance** to **Transitional Stance**. Stand with feet shoulder-width apart. The knees are flexed at 10-20 degrees. Shift your body weight to the right leg. Lift the left heel up and get ready to step out.

Photo #2: Take a step out leftward with your left foot when you are raising your hands through the midline (**Movement 1**). The toes of the left foot are touching the ground, and the hands are at shoulder level. **Inhale** while raising the hands.

Photo #3: Gradually shift your body weight to the left leg while continuing circling your hands up. At this moment, the body weight is evenly distributed between your legs.

Photo #4: As your hands are raised overhead, about 70 percent of the bodyweight has moved to the left leg. Keep your feet in complete contact with the ground. You are in a sideward bow stance: the left knee is mildly flexed, and the right knee is straight. Your palms face forward.

Photo #5: Lower your hands without moving your feet. Namely, you remain in the sideward bow stance. Gradually turn your head toward the left. **Exhale** while lowering the hands.

Photo #6: Your arms are fully extended and stretched out at shoulder level with the palms facing down and your head facing leftward. Hold this pose for one breath or as long as you like. This pose looks like **Warrior 2 Pose** in yoga except that your stance is higher, and the tips of both feet are pointed forward.

Hereafter, **inhale** and slowly rotate your arms to turn the palms upward (supinate) while keeping stretching out your arms.

Photo #7: The palms have been turned to face upward. Next, **exhale** and circle your hands down to the sides while turning your palms downward.

Photo #8: Shift your weight back to the right leg while dropping your hands and returning your head to the front. In the meanwhile, pronate your arms so that your palms face downward. You are ready to move your left foot back to the starting location.

Photo #9: Move your left foot closer to the right foot as your hands are returning to your sides. Gradually shift your body weight to the left leg. At this moment, the body weight is evenly distributed between both legs. You are back to **Routine Stance**. You can perform the same movement by stepping out to the right with your right foot

Breathing Coordination
Photos #1, **#2,** and **#3**: Inhale while raising the hands.
Photos #4 and **#5**: Exhale while lowering the hands.

141

Photo #6: Inhale while turning the palms upward (supinate).

Photos #7 and #8: Exhale while dropping the hands and turning the palms downward (pronate).

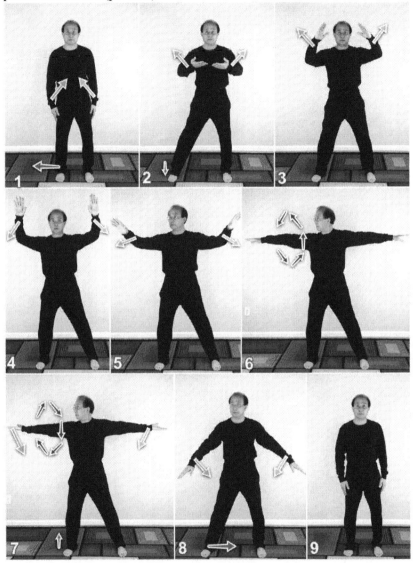

Figure 5-2C. Standing Sideward Movement 1. Take a side step with the **right foot** while performing Movement 1.

Standing Sideward Movement 2

The yoga component of this posture is derived from **Mountain Pose** variations. Please review the execution of **Movement 2** in Chapter 4.

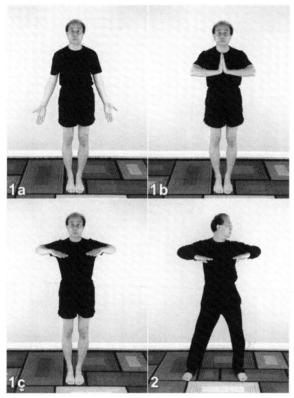

Figure 5-2D. Photo #1a, **Mountain Pose**. Photo #1b, **Mountain Pose** variation. **Photos #1c**. Chest-opening pose. Stand with your big toes touching and your heels slightly apart. Open the chest and stretch the shoulders. Spread out your arms to the sides at shoulder level with your elbows bent and palms facing downward.

Photo #2. The yoga component of **Sideward Movement 2**. Stand with your feet one to two feet apart and pointed forward. The front knee (the left knee in the figure) is mildly bent, and the back knee is straight. Both feet are in complete contact with the floor. Spread out arms to the sides with your elbows bent and your palms facing downward. Your arms are parallel to the floor. Keep your eyes looking toward the left side. See the following detailed instructions on how to perform Standing Sideward Movement 2.

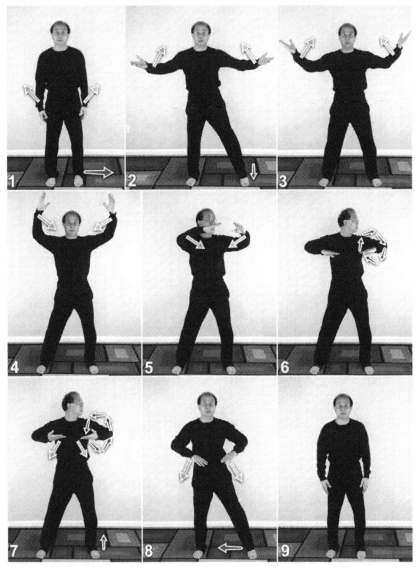

Figure 5-2E. Standing Sideward Movement 2. Take a side step with the left foot while performing Movement 2.

Key points for **Figure 5-2E**.

Photo #1: **Routine Stance** to **Transitional Stance**. Stand with feet shoulder-width apart and the knees flexed at 10-20 degrees. Shift your body weight to the right leg. Lift the left heel up and get ready to step out.

144

Photo #2: Take a step out leftward with your left foot when you are raising your hands to the sides (**Movement 2**). The toes of the left foot are touching the ground, and the hands are at shoulder level. **Inhale** while raising the hands.

Photo #3: Gradually shift your body weight to the left leg while continuing circling your hands up. At this moment, the body weight is evenly distributed between your legs.

Photo #4: As your hands are raised overhead, about 70 percent of the bodyweight has moved to the left leg. Keep your feet in complete contact with the ground. You are in a sideward bow stance: the left knee is mildly flexed, and the right knee is straight. Your palms face forward.

Photo #5: Circle your hands down through the midline without moving your feet. Namely, you remain in the sideward bow stance. Gradually turn your head toward the left. **Exhale** while lowering the hands.

Photo #6: Hold your arms at shoulder level with your elbows bent and your palms facing downward. Pull your shoulders back and open your chest with your head facing leftward. Hold this pose for one breath or as long as you like. This pose looks like a **Mountain Pose variation** in yoga except that you are in the sideward bow stance.

Hereafter, **inhale** and slowly rotate your arms to turn the palms upward (supinate) while keeping opening up your chest.

Photo #7: The palms have been turned to face upward. Next, **exhale** and circle your hands down while turning your palms downward.

Photo #8: Shift your weight back to the right leg while dropping your hands and returning your head to the front. In the meanwhile, pronate your arms so that your palms face downward. You are ready to move your left foot back to the starting location.

Photo #9: Move your left foot closer to the right foot as your hands are returning to your sides. Gradually shift your body weight back to the left leg. At this moment, the body weight is evenly distributed between both legs. You are back to **Routine Stance**. You can perform the same movement by stepping out to the right with your right foot

Breathing Coordination

Photos #1, **#2**, and **#3**: Inhale while raising the hands.

Photos #4 and **#5**: Exhale while lowering the hands.

145

Photo #6: Inhale while turning the palms upward (supinate).

Photos #7 and **#8**: Exhale while dropping the hands and turning the palms downward (pronate).

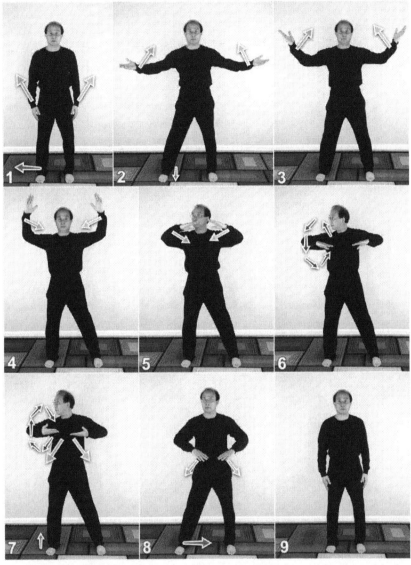

Figure 5-2F. Standing Sideward Movement 2. Take a side step with the **right foot** while performing Movement 2.

Standing Sideward Movement 3

The yoga component of this posture is derived from **Archer Pose**. Please review the execution of **Movement 3** in Chapter 4.

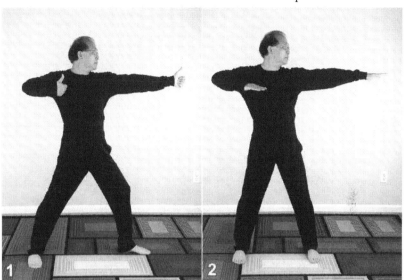

Figure 5-2G.

Photo #1: **Archer Pose**. Extend the front arm forward parallel to the ground. The back arm is bent at the elbow and pulled back at shoulder level. Make fists with the thumbs pulled back. Gaze over the thumb of your front hand. Bend the front knee so that the thigh is as close to parallel to the ground as possible. The front knee is directly over the front ankle. The back foot is turned in approximately 60-90 degrees, and the tip of the front foot is pointed leftward. The heel of the front foot is aligned with the heel or the arch of the back foot.

Photo #2: The yoga component of **Sideward Movement 3**. Stand with your feet one to two feet apart and pointed forward. The front knee (the left knee in the figure) is mildly bent, and the back knee is straight. Both feet are in complete contact with the floor. Spread out the front arm to the side with the elbow fully extended. Hold the back arm that is bent at the elbow. Your arms are parallel to the floor at shoulder level. Both palms are facing downward. Keep your eyes looking over the mid-finger of the front hand. See the following detailed instructions on how to perform Sideward Movement 3.

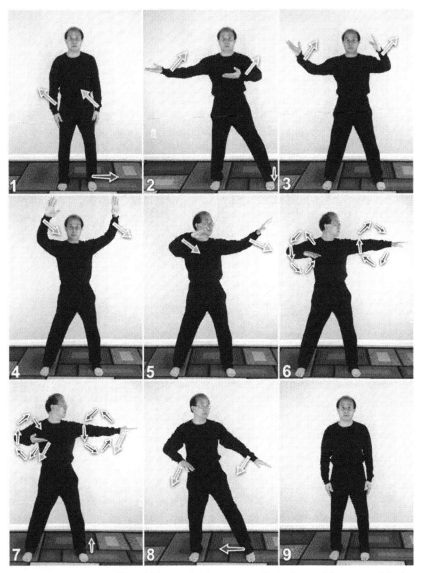

Figure 5-2H. Standing Sideward Movement 3. Take a side step with the left foot while performing Movement 3.

Key points for **Figure 5-2H**:

Photo #1: **Routine Stance** to **Transitional Stance**. Stand with feet shoulder-width apart. The knees are flexed at 10-20 degrees. Shift your body weight to the right leg. Lift the left heel up and get ready to step out.

Photo #2: Take a step sideward left when you are circling your hands counterclockwise (**Movement 3**). The toes of the left foot are touching the ground, and the hands are at shoulder level. **Inhale** while raising the hands.

Photo #3: Gradually shift your body weight to the left leg while keeping raising your hands. At this moment, the body weight is evenly distributed between both legs.

Photo #4: As your hands are raised overhead, about 70 percent of the bodyweight has moved to the left leg. Keep your feet in complete contact with the ground. You are in a sideward bow stance: the left knee is mildly flexed, and the right knee is straight. Your palms face forward.

Photo #5: Circle your hands down without moving your feet. Namely, you remain in the sideward bow stance. Gradually turn your head toward the left. **Exhale** while lowering the hands.

Photo #6: Your left arm is fully extended, and the bent right arm is held at shoulder level. At this time, the palms face downward, and the head faces leftward. Hold this pose for one breath or as long as you like. This pose looks like **Archer Pose** in yoga and many postures in qigong.

Hereafter, **inhale** and slowly rotate your arms to turn the palms upward (supinate) while keeping stretching out your arms.

Photo #7: The palms have been turned to face upward. Next, **exhale** and circle your hands down while turning your palms downward.

Photo #8: Shift your weight back to the right leg while dropping your hands and returning your head to the front. In the meanwhile, pronate your arms so that your palms face downward. You are ready to move your left foot back to the starting location.

Photo #9: Move your left foot closer to the right foot as your hands are returning to your sides. Gradually shift your body weight back to the left leg. At this moment, the body weight is evenly distributed between both legs. You are back to **Routine Stance**. You can perform the same movement by stepping out to the right with your right foot

Breathing Coordination

Photos #1, #2, and **#3**: Inhale while raising the hands.

Photos #4 and **#5**: Exhale while lowering the hands.

Photo #6: Inhale while turning the palms upward (supinate).

Photos #7 and **#8**: Exhale while dropping the hands and turning the palms downward (pronate).

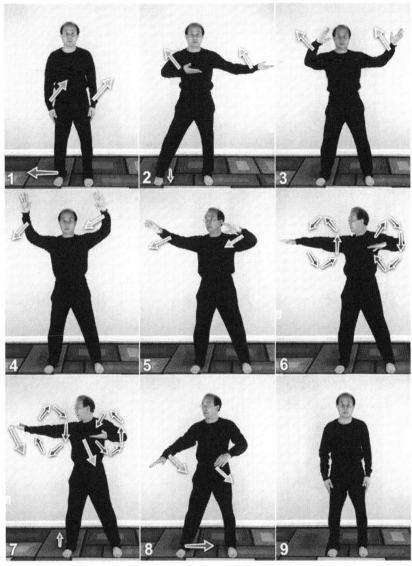

Figure 5-2I. Standing Sideward Movement 3. Take a side step with the **right foot** while performing Movement 3.

Downward and Backward Postures

Standing Downward Movement 2

The yoga component of this posture is derived from **Standing Forward Bend** (Uttanasana). Please review the execution of **Movement 2** in Chapter 4.

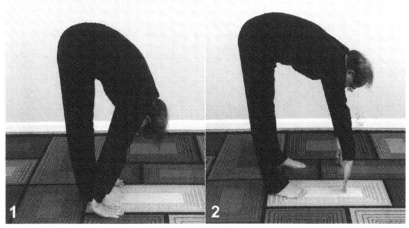

Figure 5-3A.

Photo #1: **Standing Forward Bend** (Uttanasana). Stand with your big toes touching and your heels slightly apart. Fold your torso over your legs at the hips with the knees straight or slightly flexed. The palms rest on either side of your feet on the floor. Bend your knees more if you cannot touch the floor. If you have difficulty maintaining balance, stand with your feet shoulder-width apart.

Photo #2: The yoga component of **Downward Movement 2**. Stand with your feet shoulder-width apart and your knees straight or slightly flexed. Bend forward at the hips with your fingers or palms touching the floor in front of the feet. See the following detailed instructions on how to perform **Downward Movement 2**.

Cautions and Contraindications: back or neck pain/injury, dizziness, glaucoma, and cardiovascular diseases.

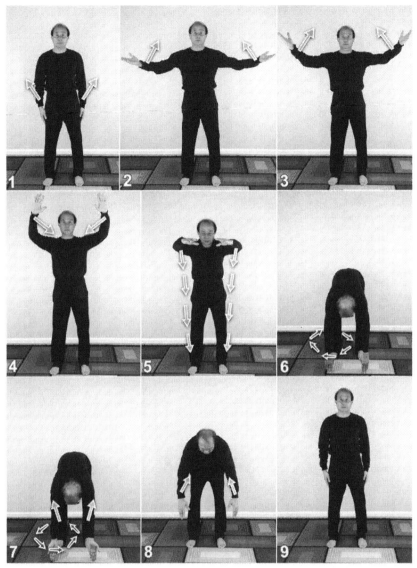

Figure 5-3B. Standing Downward Movement 2 (front view).

Key points for **Figure 5-3B** and **Figure 5-3C**.

Photo #1: Start with **Routine Stance**. Stand with feet shoulder-width apart. The knees are flexed at 10-20 degrees.

Photo #2: Slowly straighten your knee joints when you are raising your hands to the sides (**Movement 2**). As the arms rotate out, the palms turn progressively and face upward. **Inhale** while raising the hands. The hands are at shoulder level at this moment.

Photo #3: The hands continue to ascend with the palms facing upward. The palms face inward as the hands are raised above shoulder level.

Photo #4: Raise your hand overhead, or to any height you like with the palms facing forward. From now, slowly bend forward at the hips.

Photo #5: You are bending forward as the hands are descending through the midline of the body. **Exhale** while lowering the hands.

Photo #6: Lower your body as far as you can with the palms facing downward and backward. Keep your knees straight if you are flexible. Otherwise, gently bend your knees and drop your hands to whatever level is comfortable for you. This pose looks like **Standing Forward Bend**. Hold the pose as long as you like.

Hereafter, **inhale** while turning your palms forward (supinate).

Photo #7: Your palms have been turned forward.

Next, **exhale** and raise your body while turning the palms backward (pronate).

Photo #8: Gradually raise your body with the palms facing backward and the knees gently flexed. Continue to exhale until you resume the upright position.

Photo #9: As you resume the upright position, your hands have returned to your sides. You are back to **Routine Stance**.

Breathing Coordination.

Photos #1, #2, and **#3**: Inhale while raising the hands.

Photos #4 and **#5**: Exhale while lowering the hands.

Photo #6: Inhale while turning the palms forward (supinate).

Photos #7 and **#8**: Exhale while turning the palms backward (pronate) and returning to the upright position.

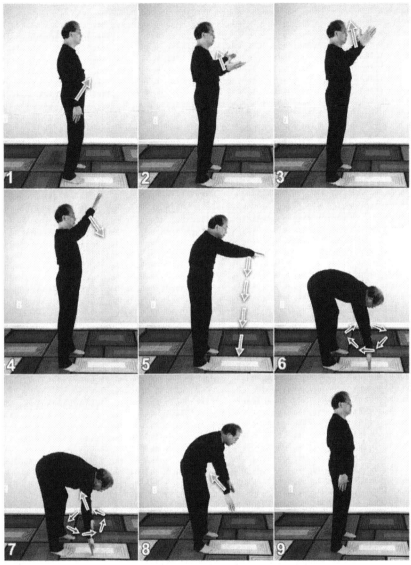

Figure 5-3C. Standing Downward Movement 2 (lateral view).

The Important Point

Do not bend at all or bend forward to a lesser degree if you have certain health conditions like back or neck pain/injury, dizziness, glaucoma, and cardiovascular diseases. See **Figure 5-3D**.

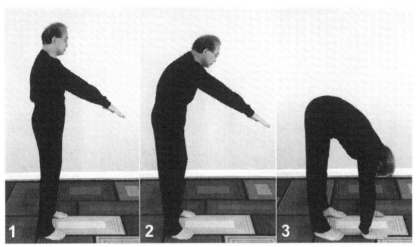

Figure 5-3D. Variations of Forward Bending.

Photo #1: Do not bend at all.

Photo #2: Bend forward to a lesser degree.

Photo #3: Touch your palms on the floor and keep your knees straight if you have good flexibility.

Standing Backward Movement 2

The yoga component of this posture is derived from **Raised Arms Pose** (Hasta Uttanasana). Please review the execution of **Movement 2** in Chapter 4.

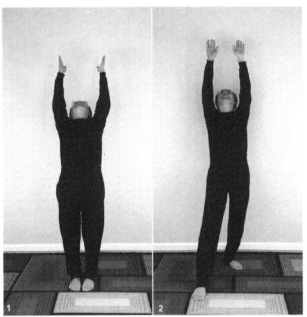

Figure 5-3E.

Photo #1. Raised Arms Pose (Hasta Uttanasana). Stand with your feet placed close to each other. Raise both your hands over the head. Keep the hands shoulder-width apart with the palms facing each other. Bend the upper body and head backward as far as you can.

Photo #2. The yoga component of **Backward Movement 2**. Take a step backward and stand with the rear leg supporting the entire weight of the body. Both feet are in complete contact with the ground. Raise your hands overhead with your elbows fully extended and your palms facing forward. Gently tilt the upper body and head backward. Keep your eyes looking forward or upward. See the following detailed instructions on how to perform **Backward Movement 2**.

Cautions and Contraindications: Dizziness, imbalance, and neck or back injury.

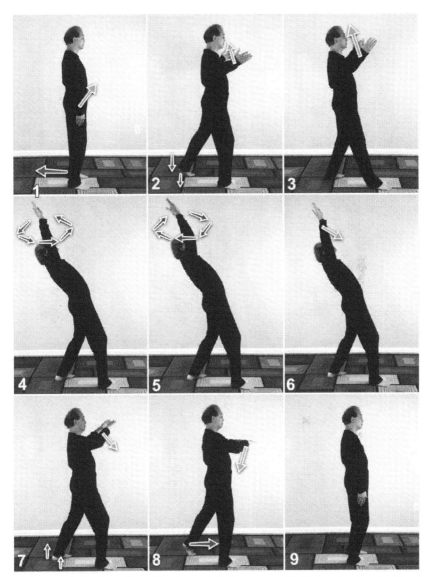

Figure 5-3G. Standing Backward Movement 2 (lateral view). Step backward with the left foot and perform Movement 2.

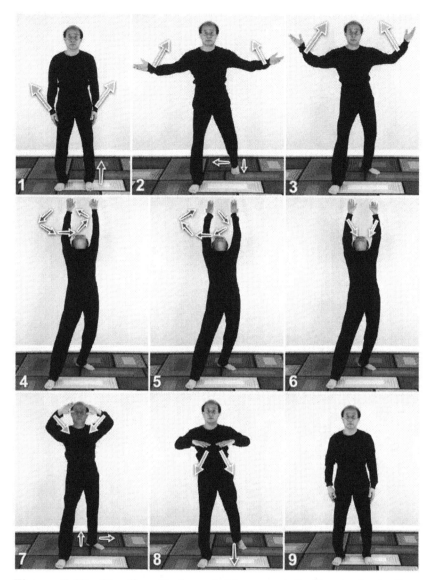

Figure 5-3F. Standing Backward Movement 2 (front view). Step backward with the left foot and perform Movement 2.

Key points for **Figure 5-3F** and **Figure 5-3G**.

Photo #1: Start with **Routine Stance**. Stand with feet shoulder-width apart and the knees flexed at 10-20 degrees. Shift the weight to the right leg and be back in **Transitional Stance** with the right leg supporting the body. You are ready to step back with your left foot.

Photo #2: Step backward with your left foot while circling your hands up to your sides (**Movement 2**). As the toes of your left foot are touching the ground, gradually shift the weight to the left leg. At this time, your hands are at shoulder level. **Inhale** while raising your hands.

Photo #3: Continue to circle your hands up and shift your weight to the left leg. As the left foot makes full contact with the ground, the left heel is naturally moved inward. At this moment, the toes of the right foot (the front foot) are pointed forward, and the left foot (the rear foot) is angled outward at 35-45 degrees.

Photo #4: Raise your hands overhead until the arms are fully extended. Gently tilt the upper body and head backward. Keep your eyes looking upward with the palms directed forward. Both feet are in complete contact with the ground. This pose looks like **Raised Arms Pose** in yoga and many postures in qigong. Hold this pose for one breath or as many breaths as you like.

Hereafter, **exhale,** and slowly rotate your arms to turn the palms backward (supinate).

Photo #5: Your palms have been turned backward while staying in the pose. Next, **inhale** and rotate your arms to turn the palms forward again (pronate).

Photo #6: Your palms have been turned forward. Then, straighten the trunk and shift the weight back to the right leg (the front leg). At the same time, circle your hands down through the midline of the body and turn the palms downward (pronate). **Exhale** slowly when dropping your hands with the palms facing downward.

Photo #7: Your arms are above shoulder level, and the bodyweight is moving gradually to the right leg with the trunk straightening.

Photo #8: As the weight has shifted to the right leg, the left heel is raised off the ground and spontaneously moved outward with the tip of the left foot pointed forward. Your hands have descended to shoulder level at this moment. You are ready to step forward with the left foot.

Photo #9: Step forward with the left foot and position the left foot parallel to the right foot. Shift your weight to the left leg and return your hands to your sides. At this moment, the weight is evenly distributed between two legs. Now you are back in **Routine Stance** and are ready to go on to the next posture.

Breathing Coordination. Photos #1, #2, and **#3**: Inhale while raising the hands. **Photo #4**: Exhale while turning the palms backward (supinate). **Photo #5**: Inhale while turning the palms forward (pronate). **Photos #6, #7,** and **#8**: Exhale while lowering the hands.

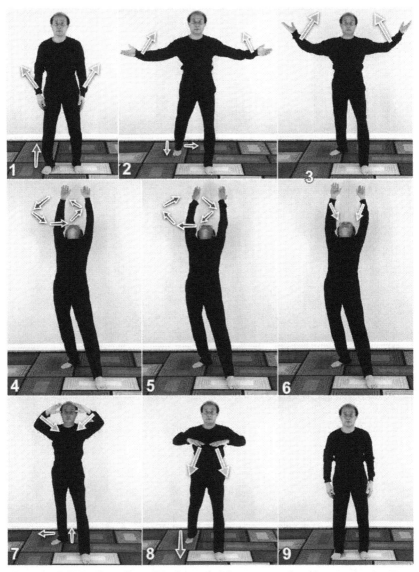

Figure 5-3H. Standing Backward Movement 2. (front view). Step backward with the **right foot** and perform Movement 2.

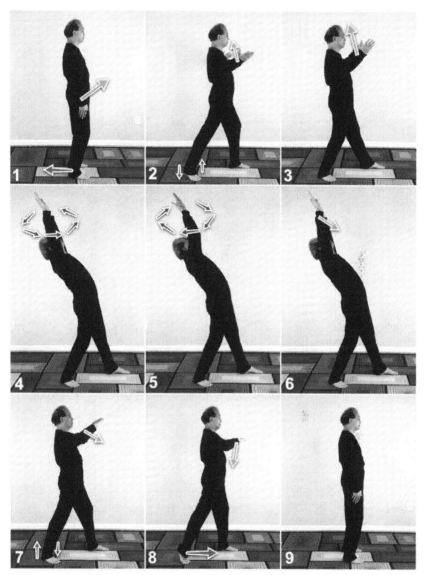

Figure 5-3I. Standing Backward Movement 2 (lateral view). Step backward with the **right foot** and perform Movement 2.

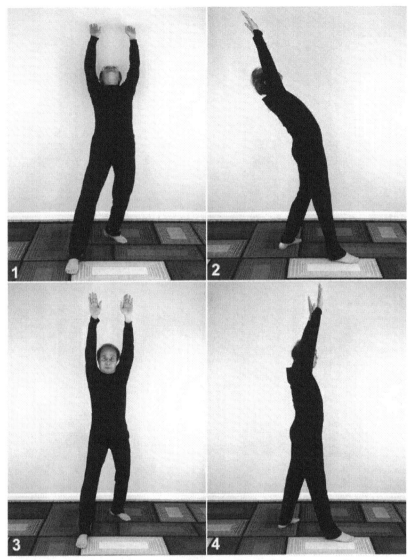

Figure 5-3J. Variations of Standing Backward Movement 2.

The Important Point

Photos #1 and **#2**: Bend backward as far as you feel comfortable.

Photos #3 and **#4**: Bend backward to a lesser degree or do not bend at all if you have certain health conditions like neck/back pain, dizziness, imbalance, etc.

Raise your hands to any height that is comfortable for you if you have shoulder pain or injury.

Balance Postures

These balance postures are similar to **Tree Pose** and its variations in yoga. Principally, raise one of your legs when you circle your hands up and drop the leg back to the ground when circling your hands down. If you have trouble balancing, do not lift your leg too high or do not lift your leg at all.

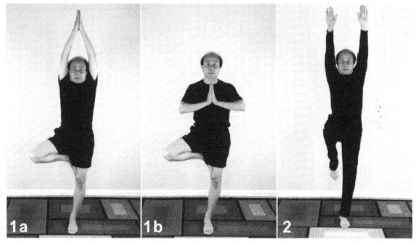

Figure 5-4A. **Tree Pose**, its variation, and a balance posture in Yoga E Tai Chi.

Photo #1a: **Tree Pose** (Vriksasana), an essential pose in yoga. Draw and press one of your feet (the right foot in the figure) into your left inner thigh. Raise your hands overhead with your elbows fully extended and your palms pressed together. Look straight ahead in front of you.

Photo #1b: A **Tree Pose** variation. Press your palms together in Namaste mudra.

Photo #3: The yoga component of **Balance Movement 1a**. Lift one leg (the right leg in the figure) with the knee bent as high as you can and hold it as you raise your hands overhead. Keep the knee of the supporting leg (the left leg in the figure) straight. The palms are directed forwards.

Balance Movement 1a

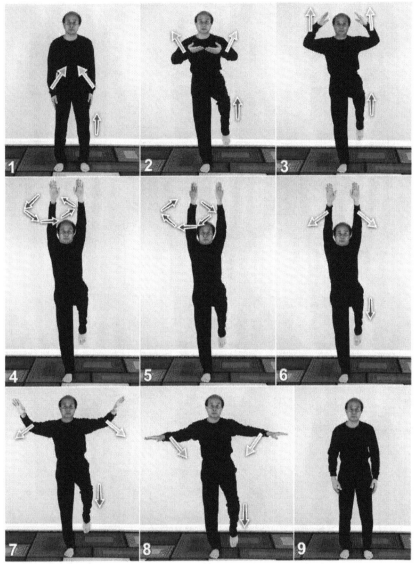

Figure 5-4B. Balance Movement 1a. Lift the left leg and perform Movement 1.

Key points for **Figure 5-4B.**

Photo #1: **Routine Stance**. Stand with feet shoulder-width apart. Your hands rest at your sides. The knees are flexed at 10-20 degrees. Keep your torso upright.

Photos #2: Shift your weight to the right leg and gradually lift your left leg with the knee bent. Slowly straighten your right knee when you are raising your hands along the midline (**Movement 1**). The palms are directed upward when the hands are ascending. The fingers of both hands point to each other diagonally. You look like you are holding a big ball in front of your body. **Inhale** while raising the hands.

Photo #3: When your hands are raised above shoulder level, your palms gradually turn (pronate) to face inward during the transition from facing upward to facing forward. Continue to lift your left leg.

Photo #4: As your hands are raised overhead and fully extended, the palms are directed forwards, and the right knee is straight. Keep your eyes looking forward or upward. With the knee bent, lift your left leg as high as you can and hold it. This pose looks like **Tree Pose**. Hold the pose for one breath or as many breaths as you like.

Hereafter, **exhale** and slowly rotate your arms to turn the palms backward (supinate) while keeping your arms straightened.

Photo #5: Your palms have been turned to face backward. Next, **inhale** and rotate your arms to turn the palms forward (pronate).

Photo #6: Your palms have been turned to face forward. From now, lower your arms and your left leg while slowly flexing your right knee.

Photo #7: Slowly drop your arms while turning the palms downward (pronate). Gently bend your right knee and lower your left leg. Exhale while lowering your hands.

Photo #8: At this moment, the hands are at shoulder level with the palms facing downward. The left leg and the hands continue to descend.

Photo #9: The hands have returned to your sides, and the left foot has come in complete contact with the ground. The knees are gently flexed. You are back to **Routine Stance** and ready to perform the next posture: raise your **right** leg and perform the same hand movement described above.

Breathing Coordination. Photos #1, **#2**, and **#3**: Inhale while raising the hands. **Photo #4**: Exhale while turning the palms backward (supinate). **Photo #5**: Inhale while turning the palms forward (pronate). **Photos #6**, **#7**, and **#8**: Exhale while lowering the hands.

Balance Movement 1b

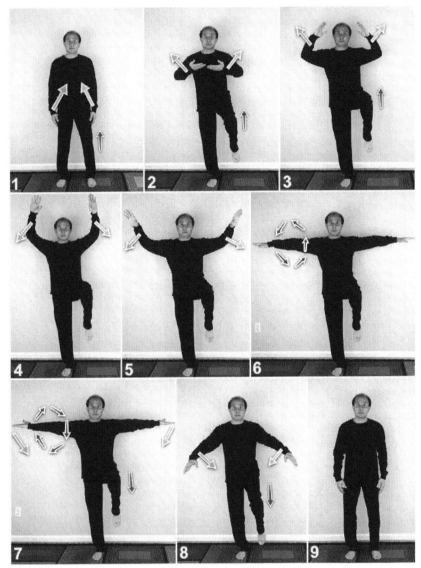

Figure 5-4C. Balance Movement 1b. Lift the left leg and perform Movement 1.

Key points for **Figure 5-4C.**

Photo #1: **Routine Stance**. Stand with feet shoulder-width apart. Your hands rest at your sides. The knees are flexed at 10-20 degrees. Keep your torso upright.

Photos #2: Shift your weight to the right leg and gradually lift your left leg with the knee bent. Slowly straighten your right knee when you are raising your hands along the midline (**Movement 1**). The palms are directed upward when the hands are ascending. The fingers of both hands point to each other diagonally. You look like you are holding a big ball in front of your body. **Inhale** while raising the hands.

Photo #3: When your hands are raised above shoulder level, your palms gradually turn (pronate) to face inward during the transition from facing upward to facing forward. Continue to lift your left leg.

Photo #4: Your hands are raised overhead with the right knee straight and the palms directed forwards. With the left knee bent, lift your left leg as high as you can and hold it.

Photo #5: **Exhale** while lowering your hands to the sides and holding your left leg up.

Photo #6: Your arms are fully extended at shoulder level with the palms facing down. Hold this pose for one breath or as long as you like. This pose looks like **Tree Pose** plus **Warrior 2 Pose**.

Hereafter, **inhale** and slowly rotate your arms to turn the palms upward (supinate) while keeping stretching out your arms.

Photo #7: Your palms have been turned to face upward. Next, lower your arms and your left leg and gently flex your right knee. **Exhale** while turning the palms downward and dropping your hands.

Photo #8: Continue to lower the left leg and flex the right knee while dropping your hands with the palms facing downward.

Photo #9: Your hands have returned to your sides with the knees gently flexed. You are back to **Routine Stance** and ready to perform the next posture: raise your **right** leg and perform the same hand movement described above.

Breathing Coordination

Photos #1, #2, and **#3**: Inhale while raising the hands.

Photos #4 and **#5**: Exhale while lowering the hands.

Photo #6: Inhale while turning the palms upward (supinate).

Photos #7 and **#8**: Exhale while dropping the hands and turning the palms downward (pronate).

Balance Movement 2

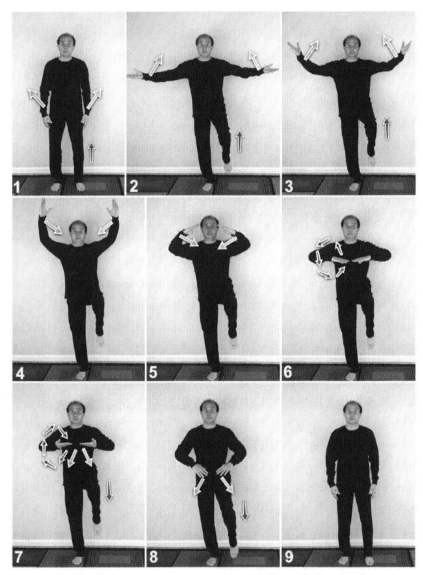

Figure 5-4D. Balance Movement 2. Lift the left leg and perform Movement 2.

Key points for **Figure 5-4D.**

Photo #1: **Routine Stance**. Stand with feet shoulder-width apart. Your hands rest at your sides. The knees are flexed at 10-20 degrees. Keep your torso upright.

Photos #2: Shift your weight to the right leg and gradually lift your left leg with the knee bent. Slowly straighten your right knee when you are circling your hands up to the sides (**Movement 2**) with the palms facing upward. **Inhale** while raising the hands.

Photo #3: The hands continue to ascend. The palms face inward as the hands are raised above shoulder level. Keep lifting your left leg at this moment.

Photo #4: Your hands are raised overhead with the right knee straight and the palms directed forwards. With the left knee bent, lift your left leg as high as you can and hold it.

Photo #5: **Exhale** and lower your hands through the midline while holding your left leg up.

Photo #6: Your arms are held at shoulder level with the elbows bent and the palms facing down. Stay in this pose for one breath or as long as you like. This pose likes a **Tree Pose** variation.

Hereafter, **inhale** and slowly rotate your arms to turn the palms upward (supinate).

Photo #7: Your palms have been turned to face upward. Next, lower the left leg and gently flex the right knee while dropping your hands through the midline. In the meanwhile, pronate your arms so that your palms face downward. **Exhale** while dropping your hands.

Photo #8: Continue to lower the left leg and flex the right knee while dropping your hands with the palms facing downward.

Photo #9: Your hands have returned to your sides with the knees gently flexed. You are back to **Routine Stance** and ready to perform the next posture: raise your **right** leg and perform the same hand movement described above.

Breathing Coordination

Photos #1, #2, and #3: Inhale while raising the hands.

Photos #4 and #5: Exhale while lowering the hands.

Photo #6: Inhale while turning the palms upward (supinate).

Photos #7 and #8: Exhale while dropping the hands and turning the palms downward (pronate).

Balance Movement 3

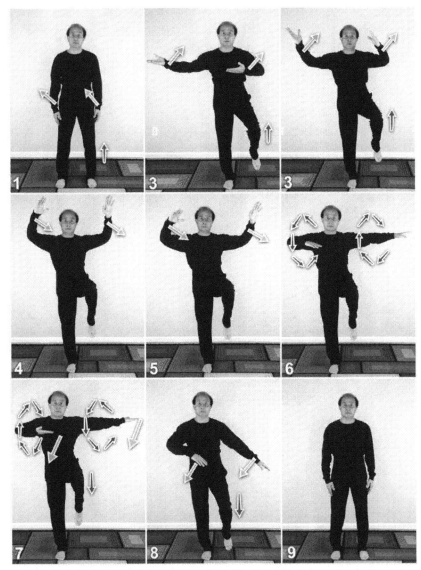

Figure 5-4E. Balance Movement 3: Lift the **left** leg and perform the **leftward** Movement 3.

Key points for **Figure 5-4E.**

Photo #1: Start with **Routine Stance**. Stand with feet shoulder-width apart. The knees are flexed at 10-20 degrees. Keep your torso upright.

Photos #2: Shift your weight to the right leg and gradually lift your left leg with the left knee bent. Slowly straighten your right knee joint while simultaneously circling your hands counterclockwise (the leftward **Movement 3**). **Inhale** while raising the hands.

Photo #3: The hands and the left leg continue to ascend.

Photo #4: Raise your hand overhead, or to any height you like with the right knee straight and the palms facing forward. Lift your left leg as far as you can and hold it.

Photo #5: **Exhale** while circling your hands down and holding your left leg up.

Photo #6: Your left arm is fully extended, and the bent right arm is held at shoulder level. At this time, the palms face downward, and the head faces forward. Hold this pose for one breath or as long as you like. This pose looks like **Tree Pose** plus **Archer Pose.**

Hereafter, **inhale,** and slowly rotate your arms to turn the palms upward (supinate).

Photo #7: The palms have been turned to face upward. Next, turn your palms downward and gently flex your right knee while circling your hands down and lowering your left leg. **Exhale** while dropping your hands.

Photo #8: Continue to lower the left leg and flex the right knee while dropping your hands and breathing out.

Photo #9: Your hands have returned to your sides with the knees gently flexed. You are back to **Routine Stance** and ready to perform the next posture: perform the **rightward** Movement 3 while lifting your **right** leg.

Breathing Coordination

Photos #1, **#2**, and **#3**: Inhale while raising the hands.

Photos #4 and **#5**: Exhale while lowering the hands.

Photo #6: Inhale while turning the palms upward (supinate).

Photos #7 and **#8**: Exhale while dropping the hands and turning the palms downward (pronate).

Yoga E Tai Chi with Weights

One of the shortcomings of traditional tai chi is a lack of upper body and aerobic exercises. You can build up your upper body/arm strength by holding dumbbells or any weights while performing E Tai Chi or Yoga E Tai Chi. Especially, Movements 1, 2, 3, 4, and 5 can be perfectly integrated into weight exercises. How much weight you want to use is up to you. I suppose 1 to 2 pounds would be a good choice for walking and 2-5 pounds for standing. Moreover, you can wear weights on your ankles if you want to strengthen your leg muscles.

You can perform all the poses described above safely and comfortably with weights on your wrists and ankles. Please see the demonstrations in **Figure 5-5A** and **Figure 5-5B**. Here, I practice balance poses with 1.5-pound (0.68 kg) wrist weights and 2.5-pound (1.14 kg) ankle weights. I do not recommend ankle weights for walking due to safety reasons. It would be safe to wear ankle weights when standing or marching in space. You are still able to maintain the smoothness and relaxation of E Tai Chi with weights on your wrists and ankles.

You can turn E Tai Chi or Yoga E Tai Chi into aerobic exercises if you perform the circular hand/arm movements at a fast pace with some weights on your wrists and ankles. You can even run in space while doing E Tai Chi Movement 4 and 5. However, you should consult your medical doctor first before starting an aerobic workout.

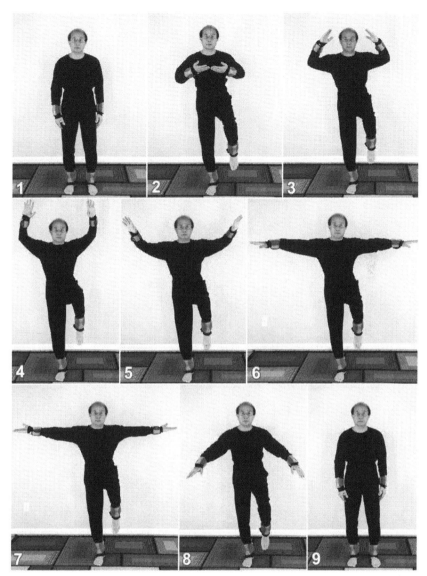

Figure 5-5A. Perform Balance Movement 1b with wrist and ankle weights.

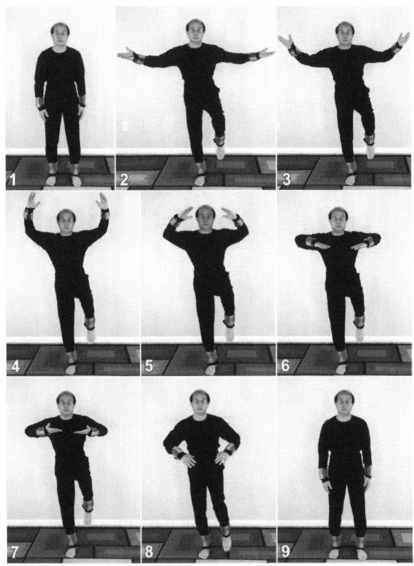

Figure 5-5B. Perform Balance Movement 2 with wrist and ankle weights.

Chapter 6. The Basic Walking Sequence in Yoga E Tai Chi

元夕

蛾儿雪柳黄金缕，笑语盈盈暗香去。

众里寻他千百度，蓦然回首，那人却在，灯火阑珊处。

The Lantern Festival Night

In gold-thread dress, with moth or willow ornaments,

Giggling, she melts into the throng with trails of scents.

But in the crowd once and again

I look for her in vain.

When all at once I turn my head,

I find her there where lantern light is dimly shed

—辛弃疾 (Xin Qiji, 1140 - 1207, Chinese poet)

Translated by 许渊冲 (Xu Yuanchong)

Megan, my daughter, standing under the lanterns in China.

When you practice a standing posture, you stand without taking a step, or you take a step with one foot and bring the foot back after finishing the posture. Specifically, you remain in the same location without moving around. During the walking sequence exercise, you just practice a series of hand/arm movements (from Movement 1 to Movement 3) continuously while walking sideways, forward, and backward. The execution of the hand movements in the walking postures is the same as in the standing postures described in the previous chapter.

It will be straightforward for you to master the basic walking sequence after you have learned the standing postures. What you need to learn is to coordinate your hand movements with your footwork. In the beginning, you can even practice the walking sequence without any coordination. Suddenly, you may find out that **Yoga E Tai Chi** is just right here and is so easy to learn after finishing this chapter. The above poem expresses the joy of discovery when it comes to yoga or tai chi learning.

Here, I use the same walking sequence for both E Tai Chi and Yoga E Tai Chi. Walk four steps sideways to the left and return to the original place. Then, walk four steps forward and walk four steps back to the starting location. However, you can take as many steps as you like. In addition, you can walk sideward to the right side instead of walking leftward. All actions are symmetrical. Do not need to twist your torso when performing Postures One, Two, and Three. **You do not need to think about the direction of palms and breathing coordination at all in the beginning. Do whatever you feel comfortable**.

If you have learned the basic E Tai Chi sequence, you can pick up the basic Yoga E Tai Chi sequence right away. You can wear weights on your wrists if you wish to intensify muscular training. Still, you can maintain the smoothness and relaxation of tai chi with weights.

The basic sequence consists of five postures plus Starting Posture and Closing Posture. They are summarized as follows:

Simplified Flow Chart for the Basic Yoga E Tai Chi Sequence

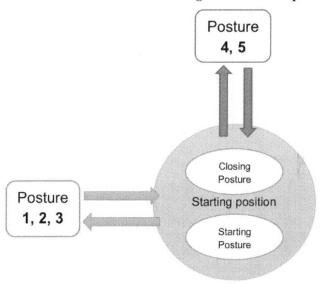

These postures are easy to remember.

Perform Standing Upward Movement 1 and Downward Movement 2 in **Starting** and **Closing Postures,** respectively.

Perform Sideward Movements **1**, **2**, and **3** while walking sideways in Postures **One**, **Two**, and **Three,** respectively.

Posture Four: perform Forward Movement 1 while walking forward.

Posture Five: perform Backward Movement 2 while walking backward.

Flow Chart for the Basic Yoga E Tai Chi Sequence

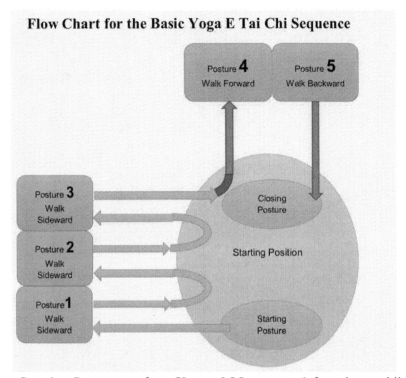

Starting Posture: perform **Upward Movement 1** four times while **standing**.

Posture **One**: perform **Sideward Movement 1** while walking 4 steps **sideways** left and 4 steps right.

Posture **Two**: perform **Sideward Movement 2** while walking 4 steps **sideways** left and 4 steps right.

Posture **Three**: perform **Sideward Movement 3** while walking 4 steps **sideways** left and 4 steps right.

Posture **Four**: perform **Forward Movement 1** while walking 4 steps **forward**.

Posture **Five**: perform **Backward Movement 2** while walking 4 steps **backward**.

Closing Posture: perform **Downward Movement 2** four times while **standing**.

Detailed Flow Chart for the Basic Yoga E Tai Chi Sequence

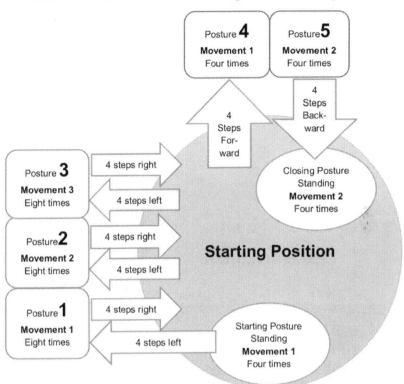

Starting Posture: perform **Upward Movement 1** four times while **standing**.

Posture **One**: perform **Sideward Movement 1** while walking 4 steps **sideways** left and 4 steps right.

Posture **Two**: perform **Sideward Movement 2** while walking 4 steps **sideways** left and 4 steps right.

Posture **Three**: perform **Sideward Movement 3** while walking 4 steps **sideways** left and 4 steps right.

Posture **Four**: perform **Forward Movement 1** while walking 4 steps **forward**.

Posture **Five**: perform **Backward Movement 2** while walking 4 steps **backward**.

Closing Posture: perform **Downward Movement 2** four times while **standing**.

Let us briefly review the basic hand/arm movements in E Tai Chi. See the details in Chapter 4.

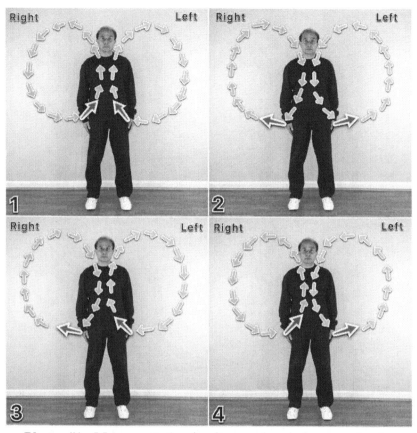

Photo #1. Movement 1: simultaneously circle your hands up through the midline of the body and circle your hands down and out to your sides (simultaneously circle your left hand counterclockwise and right hand clockwise).

Photo #2. Movement 2: simultaneously circle your hands up, out to your sides, and circle your hands down along the midline of the body (simultaneously circle your left hand clockwise and right hand counterclockwise).

Photos #3 and #4. Movement 3: simultaneously circle your hands in the same direction (counterclockwise or clockwise) in front of the body.

Starting Posture

This posture is similar to the **Commencing** posture in most of the tai chi styles and many qigong exercises. In traditional tai chi Commencing, you raise and drop your hands just in front of your torso. Your hands circle down outward to the sides of the body in Yoga E Tai Chi.

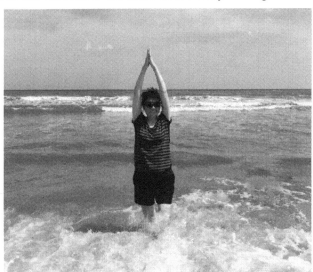

Starting Posture: Perform Upward Movement 1 **four** times while standing. This posture is exactly the same as **Standing Upward Movement 1** described in Chapter 5. Start with **Routine Stance**. Stand with your feet shoulder-width apart and your knees bent at 10-20-degrees. Keep your eyes straight ahead and breathe naturally and peacefully. See **Figure 6-1A**.

Flow Chart for Starting Postures
(Perform Movement 1 while standing.)

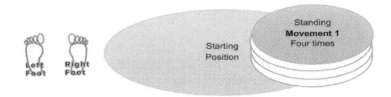

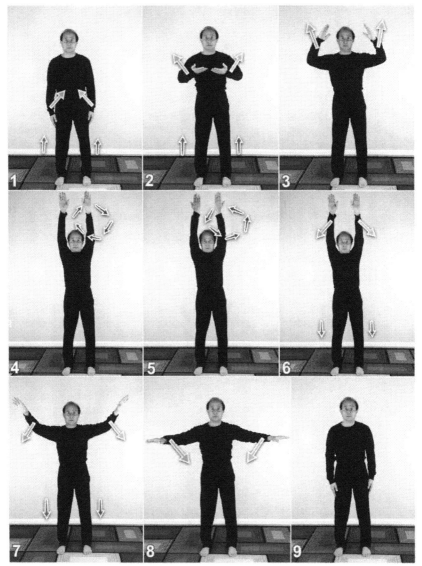

Figure 6-1A. Starting Posture: Standing Upward Movement 1 (front view).

Key points for **Figure 6-1A** and **Figure 6-1B**.

Photo #1: Routine Stance. Stand with feet shoulder-width apart. Your hands rest at your sides. The knees are flexed at 10-20 degrees. Keep your torso upright.

Photos #2: Slowly straighten your knee joints when you are raising your hands through the midline of your body (**Movement 1**). The palms are directed upward when the hands are ascending. The fingers of both hands point to each other diagonally. You look like you are holding a big ball in front of your body. **Inhale** while raising the hands.

Photo #3: When your hands are raised above shoulder level, your palms gradually turn (pronate) to face inward during the transition from facing upward to facing forward.

Photo #4: As your hands are raised overhead and fully extended, the palms are directed forwards, and the knees are straight. Keep your eyes looking forward or upward.

If you have strong legs, stand on tiptoe while holding this pose. This pose looks like **Raised Hands Pose** in yoga and many postures in qigong. Hold this pose for one breath or as many breaths as you like.

Next, **exhale** and slowly rotate your arms to turn the palms backward (supinate) while keeping your arms straightened.

Photo #5: Your palms have been turned to face backward. Hereafter, **inhale** and rotate your arms to turn the palms forward (pronate) again.

Photo #6: Your palms have been turned to face forward. From now, **exhale** while lowering your arms to the sides and turning the palms downward (pronate).

Photo #7: Drop your hands with the palms facing downward. At the same time, gradually bend your knee joints and exhale slowly.

Photo #8: At this moment, the hands are at shoulder level. The hands continue to descend with the palms facing downward.

Photo #9: The hands have returned to your sides with the knees gently flexed. You are back to **Routine Stance** and ready to perform the next posture. Repeat the above movement three more times.

Breathing Coordination.
Photos #1, **#2**, and **#3**: Inhale while raising the hands.
Photo #4: Exhale while turning the palms backward (supinate).
Photo #5: Inhale while turning the palms forward (pronate).
Photos #6, **#7**, and **#8**: Exhale while dropping the hands.

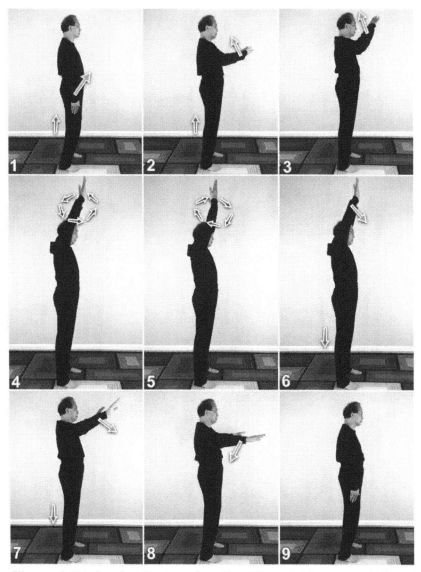

Figure 6-1B. Starting Posture: Standing Upward Movement 1 (lateral view).

The Important Point

Bend your knees to a lesser degree or do not flex your knees at all if you feel uncomfortable or pain in Routine Stance. Raise your hands to any height that is comfortable for you if you have shoulder pain or injury.

Posture One: The Sun Creeping Up

In Posture One, walk four steps sideward to the left and then walk four steps sideward right back to the starting location while doing **Sideward Movement 1**. Posture One is like the action of holding and lifting a ball. The escalating ball looks like the sun that is rising slowly.

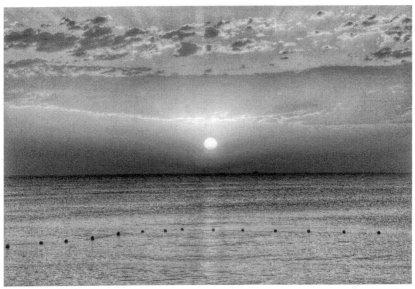

Photo provided courtesy of Xiaogang Liu.

Let us briefly review the execution of walking sideways. See the details in Chapter 3.

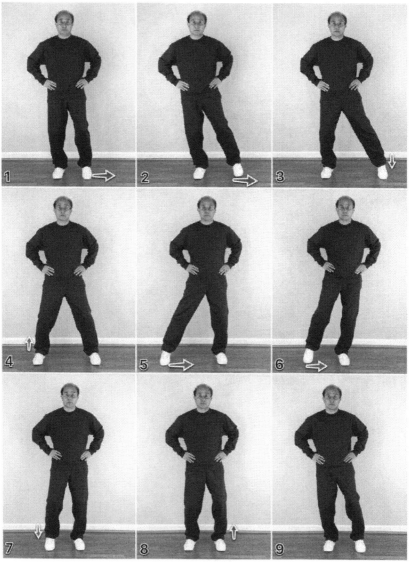

Figure 6-2A. Walking sideways (to the left).

Key points for **Figure 6-2A.**

Photo #1: **Routine Stance** to **Transitional Stance**. Stand with feet shoulder-width apart. The knees are flexed at 10-20 degrees. Keep both feet pointed forward during walking sideways. Shift your body weight to the right leg. Lift the left heel up and get ready to step out.

Photo #2: Take a step sideways left with the left foot.

Photo #3: The toes of the left foot touch the ground.

Photo #4: Gradually shift the body weight to the left leg. At this moment, the weight is evenly distributed between both legs.

Photo #5: The body weight is entirely shifted to the left leg with the right heel off the ground. You are ready to bring your right foot toward the left foot.

Photo #6: Move your right foot closer to the left foot.

Photo #7: The right foot comes in contact with the ground. The toes of the right foot touch the ground first. You are in **Transitional Stance** (the left leg is the supporting leg).

Photo #8: Gradually shift the body weight to the right leg. At this moment, the weight is evenly distributed between both legs. You are back to **Routine Stance**.

Photo #9: After having transferred your entire weight back to the right leg, you are in **Transitional Stance** again (the right leg is the supporting leg). You are ready to take the second sideward step with the left foot.

If you want to walk sideways to the right, then you can start by taking a step sideways right with the right foot in the same way as described above.

The Important Point

Bend your knees to a lesser degree or do not flex your knees at all if you feel uncomfortable or pain in Routine Stance or Transitional Stance.

Posture One: Walk **four** steps sideways to the left and perform Sideward Movement 1 **four** times, and then walk **four** steps sideways to the right and perform Sideward Movement 1 **four** times.

Flow Chart for Posture One

(Perform Movement 1 while walking sideways.)

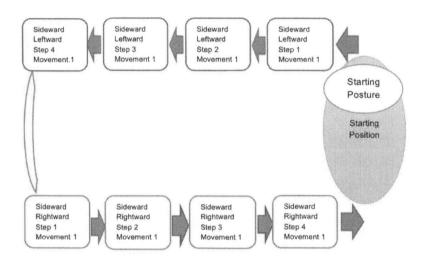

Flow Chart for Sideway Walking Steps

The numbers in the foot diagram indicate the step sequence.

The execution of Posture One.

You are in **Routine Stance** at the conclusion of Starting Posture. Stand with feet shoulder-width apart. The knees are flexed at 10-20 degrees. See **Photo #1** in **Figure 6-2B**. Shift your body weight to the right leg, and you are back in **Transitional Stance** (the right leg is the supporting leg). As you start to circle your hands up to perform Sideward Movement 1, step out to the left with your left foot. Then, gradually shift the body weight to the left leg. Be sure to make an easy sideward step. The distance between your two feet is one to two feet wide. The toes of the feet keep facing forward. See **Figure 6-2B**.

As in regular sideways walking, when you start to take a side step, lift the heel of the moving foot off the ground first and then the whole foot. The toes of the sideward-moving foot touch the ground first. The above principle applies to all the sideward-moving postures (Postures One, Two, and Three).

Breathe in when raising your hands. Shift most of your body weight to the left leg after you have raised your hands overhead or to any height you like. You are taking a sideward bow stance with the right heel raised off the ground. See **Photo #4** in **Figures 6-2B**.

Breathe out when you start to drop your arms to the sides without moving your feet. Extend your arms fully at shoulder level with your palms facing downward and gradually turn your head to the left. Hold this pose, which looks a modified **Warrior 2 Pose**. See **Photos #6** and **#7** in **Figures 6-2B** and **6-2D**.

Next, inhale and rotate your arms to turn your palms upward while staying in the pose. Then, breathe out while turning your palms downward and lowering your hands. In the meantime, move your right foot closer to the left foot. After your hands have returned to your sides with the bodyweight shifting back to the right leg, you are back to Transitional Stance and ready to execute the next posture. See **Photo #9** in **Figure 6-2B**. Repeat the same movement three more times.

After you have finished the last leftward Movement 1, simultaneously circle your hands up through the midline and walk sideways rightward back to the starting location in the same way as you do the leftward Movement 1. See **Figure 6-2D**

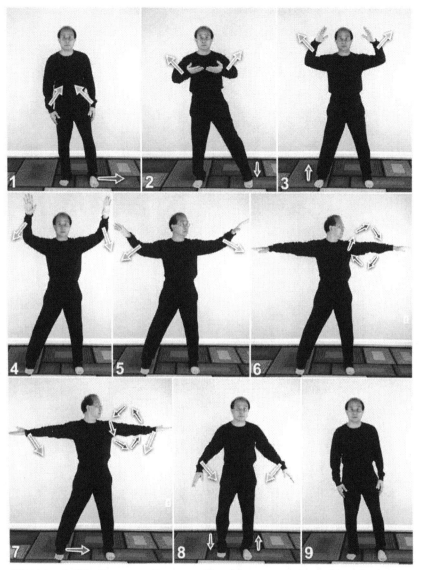

Figure 6-2B. Posture One: walk sideways leftward and perform Sideward Movement 1.

Key points for **Figure 6-2B**.

Photo #1: **Routine Stance** to **Transitional Stance**. Stand with feet shoulder-width apart. The knees are flexed at 10-20 degrees. Your hands rest at your sides. Shift your body weight to the right leg. Lift the left heel up and get ready to step out.

Photo #2: Take a step out leftward with your left foot when you are raising your hands along the midline (**Movement 1**). The toes of the left foot are touching the ground. **Inhale** while raising your hands.

Photo #3: Gradually shift your body weight to the left leg while continuing circling your hands up. At this moment, the body weight is evenly distributed between your legs.

Photo #4: As your hands are raised overhead, the body weight has moved entirely to the left leg, and the right heel comes off the ground. Your palms face forward.

Photo #5: **Exhale** while lowering your hands without moving your feet. Gradually turn your head toward the left.

Photo #6: Your arms are fully extended and stretched out at shoulder level with the palms facing down and your head facing leftward. Hold this pose for one breath or as long as you like. This pose looks like **Warrior 2 Pose** in yoga except that your stance is higher, and your right heel is lifted off the ground.

Next, **inhale** and slowly rotate your arms to turn the palms upward (supinate) while keeping stretching out your arms.

Photo #7: The palms have been turned to face upward. Hereafter, **exhale** while circling your hands down and turning your palms downward. In the meanwhile, gradually return your head to the front.

Photo #8: Move the right foot closer to the left foot while dropping your hands with the palms facing downward and the head turning toward the front. The toes of the right foot are touching the ground at this moment.

Photo #9: Gradually shift your bodyweight back to the right leg as your hands return to your sides. At this moment, you are back to **Transitional Stance** with the right leg supporting the weight and are ready to step out with the left foot again. Repeat the same movement three more times.

Breathing Coordination

Photos #1, **#2**, and **#3**: Inhale while raising the hands. **Photos #4** and **#5**: Exhale while lowering the hands. **Photos #6**: Inhale while turning the palms upward (supinate). **Photos #7** and **#8**: Exhale while dropping the hands and turning the palms downward (pronate).

There is a minor difference between the standing and walking sideward postures. See **Figure 6-2C**.

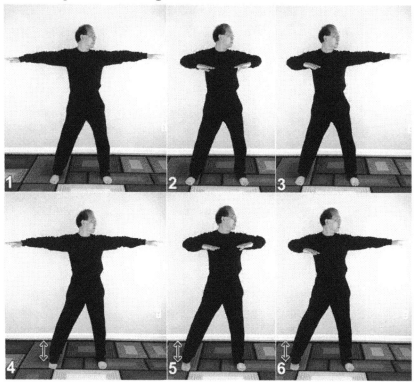

Figure 6-2C. Difference between the standing and walking sideward postures.

Photos #1, #2, and #3: In the standing sideward postures, both feet maintain full contact with the ground when you are staying in a pose. Please review Chapter 5 for details.

Photos #4, #5, and #6: In the walking sideward postures, only the toes of the rear foot (the right foot in the figure, see the arrows) touch the ground, and the front foot (here the left foot) comes in full contact with the ground while holding a pose.

You do not need to twist your torso when performing Posture One. In the beginning, you may simply walk sideways while performing hand movements without any coordination. As you have become familiar with hand/foot movements, you will coordinate your hands and feet automatically. As I said before, any coordination is fine if you feel good.

There are no absolute rules. Walk eight steps sideways in each of the sideway postures. Of course, you can take as many steps as you like.

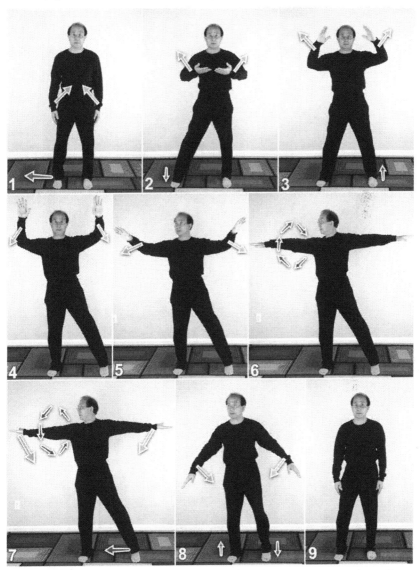

Figure 6-2D. Posture One: walk sideways **rightward** and perform Sideward Movement 1. Perform the same movement four times until you return to the starting location.

Posture Two: Seagull Flying High

In Posture Two, walk four steps sideward to the left and then walk four steps sideward right back to the starting location while doing **Sideward Movement 2**. You look like a seagull that is hovering in the sky.

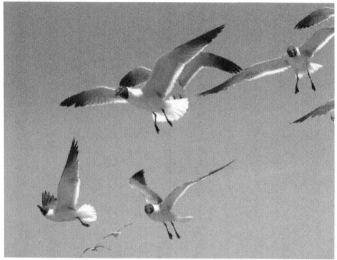

Posture Two: Walk **four** steps sideways to the left and perform Sideward Movement 2 **four** times, and then walk **four** steps sideways to the right and perform Sideward Movement 2 **four** times.

Flow Chart for Posture Two
(Perform Movement 2 while walking sideways.)

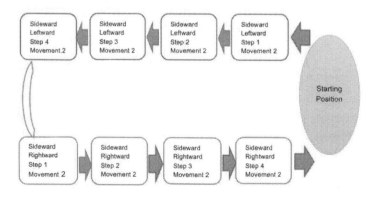

The execution of **Posture Two**.

You are back in **Transitional Stance** (the right leg is the supporting leg) after you have finished Posture One. See **Photo #1** in **Figure 6-3A**. As you start to circle your hands up to perform Sideward Movement 2, step out to the left with your left foot. Then, gradually shift your body weight to the left leg. Breathe in when raising your hands. Shift most of your body weight to the left leg after you have raised your hands overhead or to any height you like. You are taking a sideward bow stance with the right heel off the ground. See **Photo #4** in **Figure 6-3A**.

Hereafter, without moving your feet, breathe out and drop your arms through the midline while turning your head to the left. Hold your arms at shoulder level with your elbows bent and your palms facing downward. Stay in this pose, which looks a modified **Mountain Pose** or a simple chest-opening pose. See **Photos #6** and **#7** in **Figures 6-3A** and **6-3B**.

Next, inhale and rotate your arms to turn your palms upward while staying in the pose. Then, breathe out and lower your hands while turning your palms downward. In the meantime, move your right foot closer to the left foot. After your hands have returned to your sides with the bodyweight shifting back to the right leg, you are back to **Transitional Stance** and ready to execute the next posture. See **Photo #9** in **Figure 6-3A**. Repeat the same movement three more times.

Flow Chart for Sideway Walking Steps

Walking Leftward

Walking Rightward

After you have finished the last leftward Movement 2, simultaneously circle your hands up to the sides and walking sideways rightward back to the starting location in the same way as you perform the leftward Movement 2. See **Figure 6-3B**.

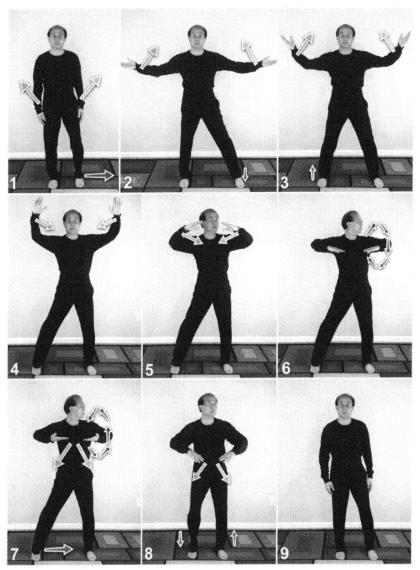

Figure 6-3A. Posture Two: walk sideways leftward and perform Sideward Movement 2.

Key points for **Figure 6-3A**.

Photo #1: **Routine Stance** to **Transitional Stance**. Stand with feet shoulder-width apart and the knees flexed at 10-20 degrees. Your hands rest at your sides. Shift your body weight to the right leg. Lift the left heel up and get ready to step out.

Photo #2: Take a step out leftward with your left foot when you are raising your hands to the sides (**Movement 2**). Right now, the toes of the left foot are touching the ground, and the arms are at shoulder level. **Inhale** while raising your hands.

Photo #3: Gradually shift your body weight to the left leg while continuing circling your hands up. At this moment, the body weight is evenly distributed between your legs.

Photo #4: As your hands are raised overhead, the body weight has been transferred to the left leg, and the right heel comes off the ground. Your palms face forward.

Photo #5: Exhale while circling your hands down through the midline without moving your feet. Gradually turn your head toward the left.

Photo #6: Your arms are held at shoulder level with the elbows bent and the palms facing down. At this moment, your head faces leftward. Pull your shoulders back and open your chest. Hold the pose for one breath or as long as you like. This pose looks like a variation of **Mountain Pose** or a simple chest-opening pose.

Next, **inhale** and slowly rotate your forearms to turn the palms upward (supinate) while holding your arms at shoulder level.

Photo #7: Your palms have been turned to face upward. Hereafter, pronate your forearms to turn your palms downward while dropping your hands. At the same time, start to **exhale** and move the right foot closer to the left foot.

Photo #8: You have moved the right foot closer to the left foot with the toes of the right foot touching the ground. In the meanwhile, drop your hands and gradually return your head to the front. Continue to exhale until your hands return to your sides.

Photo #9: Gradually shift your body weight to the right leg as your hands return to your sides. At this moment, the bodyweight has been transferred to the right leg. You are back to **Transitional Stance** and ready to step out with the left foot again. Repeat the same movement three more times.

Breathing Coordination. Photos #1, #2, and #3: Inhale while raising the hands. **Photos #4 and #5**: Exhale while lowering the hands.

Photos #6: Inhale while turning the palms upward. **Photos #7 and #8**: Exhale while dropping the hands and turning the palms downward.

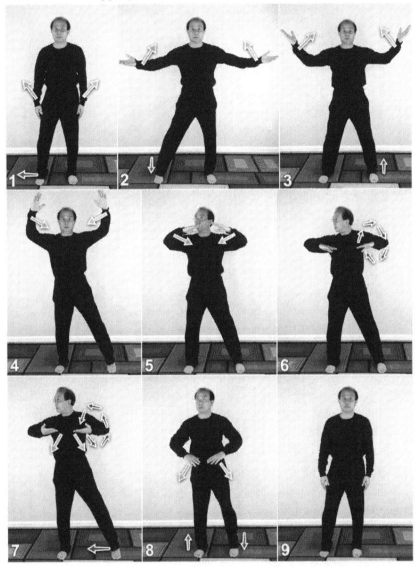

Figure 6-3B. Posture Two: walk sideways **rightward** and perform Sideward Movement 2. Perform the same movement four times until you return to the starting location.

Posture Three: Performing Yangge Dance

In Posture Three, walk four steps sideward to the left and then walk four steps sideward right back to the starting location while doing Movement 3: simultaneously circle both hands counterclockwise (to the left) and clockwise (to the right). What you are doing is like performing Yangge Dance. (For more details on this topic, see *Wikipedia: Yangge*.)

Yangge Dance is a Chinese folk dance characterized by twisting the body and waving hands rhythmically. Only Zhaobao Tai Chi has some similar movements. But the names of those movements do not fit the features of Posture Three. So, I name Posture Three "**Performing Yangge Dance**."

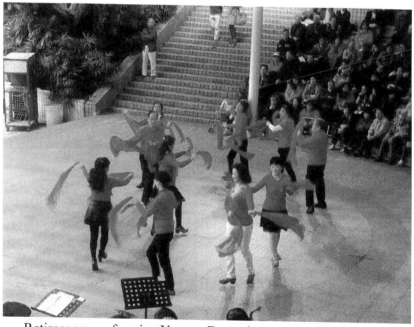

Retirees are performing Yangge Dance in Yuexiu Park in Guangzhou, China.

Posture Three: Walk **four** steps sideways to the left and perform Sideward Movement 3 **four** times, and then walk **four** steps sideways to the right and perform Sideward Movement 3 **four** times.

Flow Chart for Posture Three
(Perform Movement 3 while walking sideways.)

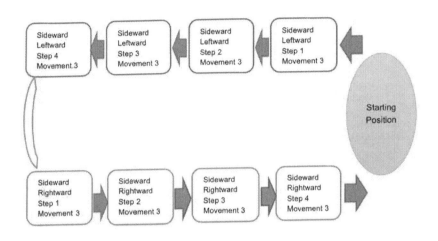

Flow Chart for Sideway Walking Steps
Walking Leftward

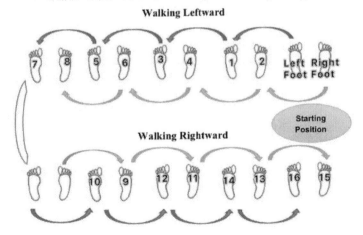

The execution of **Posture Three**.

At the conclusion of Posture Two, you are back in **Transitional Stance** (the right leg is the supporting leg). See **Photo #1** in **Figure 6-4A**. You are ready to perform leftward **Movement 3**: simultaneously circle both hands counterclockwise in front of your body. As you start to circle your hands up to perform **Movement 3**, step out to the left with your left foot. Then, gradually shift your body weight to the left leg. Breathe in when raising your hands. Shift most of your body weight to the left leg after you have raised your hands overhead or to any height you like. You are taking a sideward bow stance with the right heel off the ground. See in **Photo #4** in **Figure 6-4A**.

Without moving your feet, breathe out while dropping your arms and turning your head toward the left. Lower your arms to shoulder level with the left arm fully extended and the right elbow bent. At this moment, the palms face downward while the head faces leftward. Hereafter, stay in this pose, which looks like **Archer Pose**. See **Photos #6** and **#7** in **Figure 6-4A**.

Next, inhale and rotate your arms to turn your palms upward while staying in the pose. Then, breathe out while turning your palms downward and lowing your hands. In the meantime, move your right foot closer to the left foot and return your head to the front. After your hands have returned to your sides with the bodyweight shifting back to the right leg, you are back to **Transitional Stance** and ready to execute the next posture. See **Photo #9** in **Figure 6-4A**. Repeat the same movement three more times.

After you have finished the last leftward Movement 3, simultaneously circle your hands up clockwise and walk sideways rightward in the same way as you do the leftward Movement 3. Perform the same movement four times until you return to the starting location. See **Figure 6-4B**.

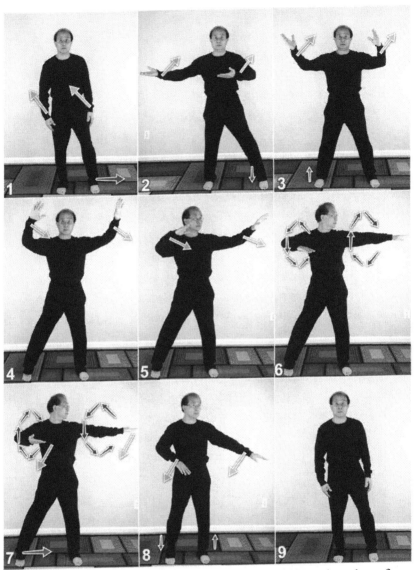

Figure 6-4A. Posture Three: walk sideways leftward and perform Sideward Movement 3.

Key points for **Figure 6-4A**:

Photo #1: At the conclusion of Posture Two, you are back in **Transitional Stance**. Standing with the right leg supporting the body and the left foot gently placed parallel to the right foot.

Photo #2: Take a step sideward left when you are circling your hands counterclockwise (**Movement 3**). **Inhale** while raising the hands. At this moment, the toes of the left foot are touching the ground, and the hands are at shoulder level.

Photo #3: Gradually shift your body weight to the left leg while keeping raising your hands. At this moment, the body weight is evenly distributed between both legs.

Photo #4: As your hands are raised overhead, the body weight has been transferred to the left leg with the right heel off the ground. Your palms face forward.

Photo #5: Without moving your feet, **exhale** while circling your hands down and turning your head toward the left.

Photo #6: Lower your hands to shoulder level with the left arm fully extended and the right elbow bent. At this moment, the palms face down while your head faces leftward. Pull your shoulders back and open your chest. Hold the pose for one breath or as long as you like. This pose looks like **Archer Pose**.

Hereafter, **inhale** and slowly rotate your forearms to turn the palms upward (supinate) while holding your arms at shoulder level.

Photo #7: Your palms have been turned to face upward. Next, pronate your forearms to turn your palms downward while circling your hands down. At the same time, start to **exhale** and move the right foot closer to the left foot.

Photo #8: You have moved the right foot closer to the left foot with the toes of the right foot touching the ground. In the meanwhile, continue to drop your hands and gradually return your head to the front. Keep breathing out until your hands return to your sides.

Photo #9: Gradually shift your body weight to the right leg as your hands return to your sides. At this moment, the bodyweight has been transferred to the right leg. You are in **Transitional Stance** again (the right leg is the supporting leg) and ready to take the second sideward step with the left foot. Repeat the same movement three more times.

Breathing Coordination. Photos #1, #2, and **#3**: Inhale while raising the hands. **Photos #4** and **#5**: Exhale while dropping the hands. **Photo #6**: Inhale while turning the palms upward (supinate). **Photos #7** and **#8**: Exhale while dropping the hands.

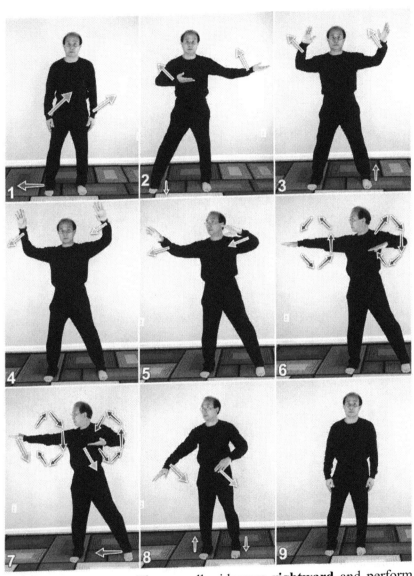

Figure 6-4B. Posture Three: walk sideways **rightward** and perform Sideward Movement 3. Perform the same movement four times until you return to the starting location.

Posture Four: Swimming on Land

Walking forward while performing Movement 1 looks like swimming breaststroke on land.

In short, when you circle your hands up, step out forward with one foot. When you drop your hands to your sides, move the other foot (the back foot) forward and place it parallel to the front foot. See the following flowchart.

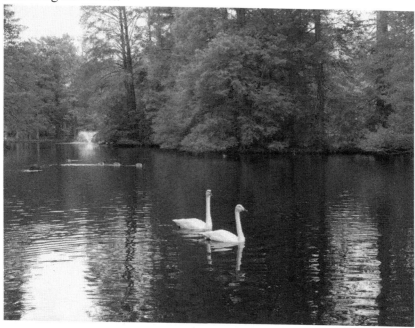

The execution of **Posture Four**. See **Figure 6-5A** and **Figure 6-5B**.

Posture Four is similar to the standing **Forward Movement 1** posture described in Chapter 4. But, in Posture Four, keep walking forward instead of staying in the same location. After having completed Posture Three, you return to your original starting position. You are back in **Transitional Stance**: the right leg is supporting the bodyweight with the toes of the left foot touching the ground. Now, you are ready to step forward with your left foot. See **Photo #1** in **Figure 6-5A**.

Posture Four: Walk **four** steps forward and perform Forward Movement 1 **four times.**

Flow Chart of Posture Four
(Perform Movement 1 while walking forward.)

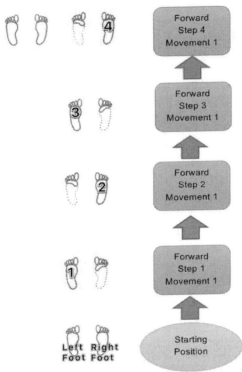

Lift your left foot and step forward while circling your arms up through the midline to perform Forward **Movement 1**. Inhale while raising your hands. As in regular walking, when you start to take a step, lift the heel of the moving foot off the ground first and then the whole foot. The heel of the forward-moving foot touches the ground first. See **Photo #2** in **Figure 6-5A**. The above principle applies to all the forward postures.

Extend your arms overhead with the palms facing forward. Keep your eyes looking forward or upward. In the meantime, gradually sink the torso and shift the body weight from the right leg to the left leg. See **Photo #3** in **Figure 6-5A**. Both feet will be in complete contact with the ground. Now you are taking a small **bow stance** with the left knee slightly bent in front and the right leg straight behind you. Seventy percent of the body weight should be distributed to the front foot and 30 % to the rear foot. This pose looks like **Warrior 1 Pose**. Stay in this pose for one breath or as many breaths as you like. See **Photos #4, #5, and #6** in **Figure 6-5A** and **Figure 6-5B**.

Hereafter, breathe out while holding the extended arms and rotating them to turn your palms backward. Then, breathe in while turning your palms forward again.

Next, breathe out and descend the hands with your palms facing downward. In the meantime, as you shift the entire body weight to the left leg (the front leg), slowly lift your right heel off the ground. When your hands are lowered to shoulder level, swing the right leg forward. See **Photos #7** and **#8** in **Figure 6-5A**. The left leg supports the whole-body weight during the swing of the right leg.

Your right foot is positioned next to the left foot as the hands return to your sides. Gently place the toes of the right foot on the ground. Now you have returned to **Transitional Stance**. See **Photo #9** in **Figure 6-5A**. Here, the left leg supports the body. Alternatively, you can skip **Transitional Stance** and continue the forward step without touching the ground if you have strong legs.

Then, go on to take the second step with the right foot while raising your hands again to perform the next Forward Movement 1. Repeat the same action as above. The difference is that you take a right forward step. See **Figure 6-5C** and **Figure 6-5D**.

In this posture, you circle your hands up and down while walking forward. You look like you are swimming breaststroke on land. Remember, it is a normal walking step at a slower pace. Your step length should be similar to the one during your normal walking. You should take comfortable steps to avoid knee pain or injury.

Repeat the left forward step and the right forward step one more time while playing Forward Movement 1. Perform Forward Movement 1 four times and take a total of four forward steps. Obviously, you can play them as many times as you like. After you have finished the last Forward Movement 1, you are back in **Transitional Stance** with the right leg supporting the body weight. Now you are ready to go on to **Posture Five**.

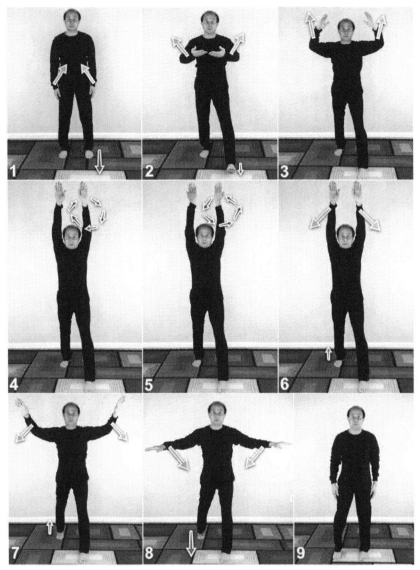

Figure 6-5A. Posture Four, the first step (front view). Walk forward and perform Forward Movement 1.

Key points for **Figure 6-5A** and **Figure 6-5B**.

Photo #1: You have completed the last rightward Movement 3 with your hands at your sides. You are in **Transitional Stance** with the right leg supporting the body weight. You are ready to step forward with the left foot.

Photo #2: Take a step forward with your left foot while circling your hands up through the midline (**Movement 1**). **Inhale** while raising the hands. At this moment, your left heel is touching the ground while your arms are at shoulder level.

Photo #3: When your hands are raised above shoulder level, your palms gradually turn (pronate) to face inward. Now, your left foot comes in complete contact with the ground.

Photo #4: Gradually shift your weight to the left leg and extend your arms overhead with the palms facing forward. Now you are taking a small **bow stance** with the left knee slightly bent in front and the right leg straight behind you. Keep your eyes looking forward or upward. This pose looks like **Warrior 1 Pose** in yoga. Hold this pose for one breath or as many breaths as you like.

When shifting the body weight from the right leg to the left leg, you should use the back leg (here the right leg) to push the body forward so that the front lower leg (here the left leg) forms a 90-degree angle relative to the ground. When **you drive the body forward by the back leg**, the front knee joint will not be over-flexed.

Next, **exhale** and slowly rotate your arms to turn the palms backward (supinate) while keeping your arms straightened.

Photo #5: Your palms have been turned to face backward. Hereafter, **inhale,** and rotate your arms to turn the palms forward (pronate) again.

Photo #6: Your palms have been turned to face forward. From now, **exhale** and lower your arms with the palms facing downward.

Photo #7: Drop your arms slowly to the sides while turning the palms downward (pronate). In the meantime, shift your entire body weight to your left leg and lift your right heel off the ground.

Photo #8: The hands continue to descend with the palms facing downward. At this moment, your hands are at shoulder level, and your weight has been completely shifted to the left leg. You are ready to swing your right foot forward.

Photo #9: Your right foot has moved forward to become parallel to the left foot. Your hands have returned to your sides with the toes of the right foot touching the ground while the left leg is supporting the body. Now you are back in **Transitional Stance** and ready to proceed to perform the next Forward Movement 1. See **Figures 6-5C** and **6-5D**.

Breathing Coordination. Photos #1, **#2**, and **#3**: Inhale while raising the hands. **Photo #4**: Exhale while turning the palms backward (supinate). **Photo #5**: Inhale while turning the palms forward (pronate). **Photos #6**, **#7**, and **#8**: Exhale while lowering the hands.

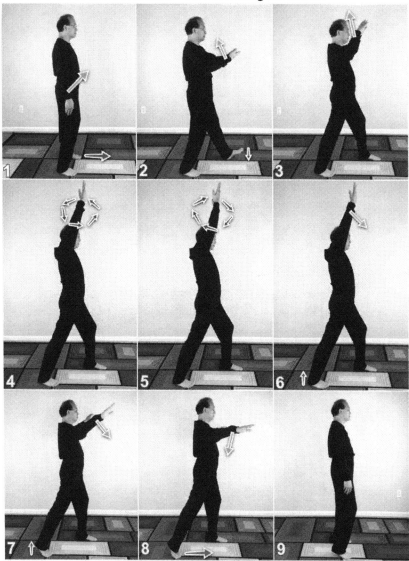

Figure 6-5B. Posture Four, the first step (lateral view).

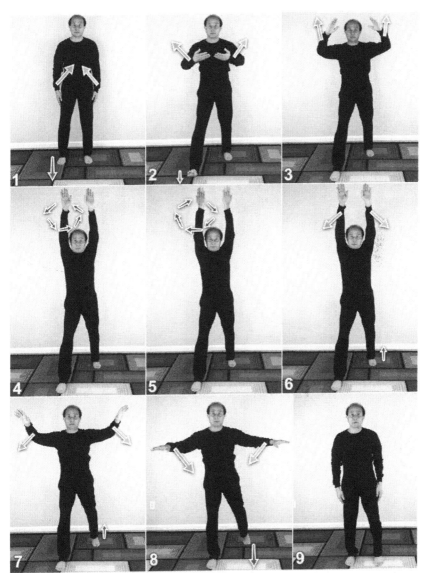

Figure 6-5C. Posture Four, the second step (front view).

Figure 6-5C and **Figure 6-5D** shows the second step in Posture Four. You do the same thing as in **Figure 6-5A** and **Figure 6-5B,** except you step forward with the right foot instead of the left foot. Repeat the same action with your left foot and right foot one more time, respectively. Walk four steps forward and perform Forward Movement 1 four times in Posture Four.

211

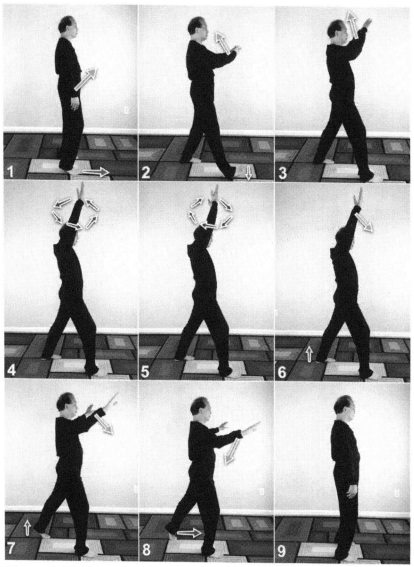

Figure 6-5D. Posture Four, the second step (lateral view).

The Important Point

Bend your front knee to a lesser degree and take shorter steps if you feel uncomfortable or pain in **Bow Stance**. Raise your hands to any height that is comfortable for you if you have shoulder pain or injury.

Posture Five: Swan Spreading Its Wings

Walking backward while performing Backward Movement 2.

This posture is similar to **White Crane Spread Its Wings** (白鶴亮翅) in many styles of tai chi, where one hand moves down to the side while another hand rises above the head. In E Tai Chi or Yoga E Tai Chi Posture Five, you imitate a swan spreading its wings because your hands ascend simultaneously.

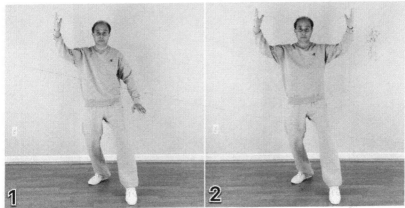

Photo #1: **White Crane Spread Its Wings** in traditional tai chi.
Photo #2: **Swan Spreading Its Wings** in E Tai Chi.

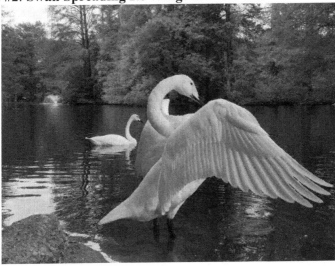

Posture Five: Walk **four** steps backward and perform Backward Movement 2 **four** times.

Flow Chart of Posture Five

(Perform Movement 2 while walking backward.)

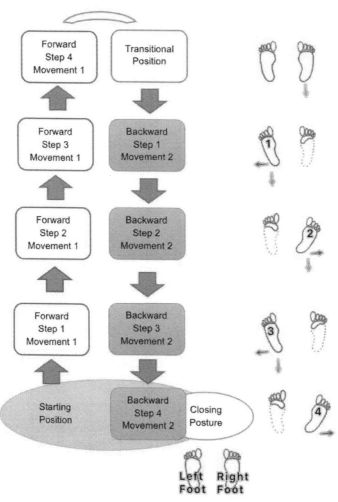

Let us practice **Posture Five**.

Posture Five is similar to the standing **Backward Movement 2** posture described in Chapter 4. But, in Posture Five, you keep walking backward instead of staying in the same location. At the conclusion of Posture Four, you are back in **Transitional Stance** with the right leg supporting the body weight. See **Photos #1** in **Figure 6-6A**. Circularly spread the hands outward (**Movement 2**) as you raise your left foot and step backward. The toes of your left foot touch the ground first. Then, the whole foot plants on the ground completely as the body weight is gradually transferred to the left leg (the rear leg). It is a natural backward step that is slowed down. Make sure not to stride too long. Otherwise, you can hurt your knee joints. Inhale while raising the hands.

As in regular backward walking, when you start to take a step backward, lift the heel of the backward-moving foot off the ground first and then the whole foot. The toes of the backward-moving foot touch the ground first. This principle applies to all the backward-moving postures.

The left heel will be naturally moved inward as the whole foot contacts the ground, and the body weight is gradually shifted to the left leg. Consequently, the left foot (the rear foot) is angled outward at 35-45 degrees. The inward movement of the heel should occur spontaneously because the resulting posture produces optimal body stability. The final posture is: the toes of the right foot (the front foot) are pointed forward, and the left foot (the rear foot) is angled outward at 35-45 degrees. See **Flowchart of Posture Five** and **Photos #2-#3** in **Figure 6-6A** and **Figure 6-6B**.

Please make sure not to let the heel of the real foot cross the midline. The crossing of your feet can easily make you lose balance. As I mentioned, you do it right when you feel natural and comfortable.

As you continue to circle your hands up above shoulder level, shift the entire body weight to the left leg. In this position, the whole body is supported by the left leg (the rear leg). Raise your hands overhead until the arms are fully extended. And gently tilt the upper body and head backward. Keep your eyes looking upward with the palms directed forwards. In the meanwhile, the right foot will move backward a few inches spontaneously. This posture happens spontaneously because it produces optimal body stability and makes you feel comfortable. Now you are in **Empty Stance**. See **Photos #4, #5**, and **#6** in **Figure 6-6A** and **Figure 6-6B**.

When your hands are raised overhead, you feel like a swan that is spreading its wings. This pose looks like **Raised Arms Pose** in yoga and many postures in qigong. Hold this pose for one breath or as many breaths as you like.

Next, slowly rotate your arms to turn the palms backward (supinate) while keeping your arms straightened. Breathe out when supinating the hands. You do not need to think about breathing coordination in the beginning. Just breathe spontaneously.

While staying in the pose, rotate your arms to turn the palms forward again (pronate). Breathe in when pronating the hands.

Then, slowly straighten your back and return to the original upright position as you are circling your hands down through the midline of the body. In the meanwhile, exhale slowly while dropping your hands with the palms facing downward. Slowly bring your right foot (the front foot) back as you continue to lower your hands.

Position your right foot next to your left foot when the hands return to your sides. Now, you are back in **Transitional Stance** with your left leg supporting the body weight. You can gently place the toes of your right foot on the ground. Alternatively, continue your backward step without touching the ground and repeat the same action as above.

Hereafter, take a step backward with the right foot. Your left foot becomes the front foot and is angled at 30-45 degrees. See **Photos #2 and #3** in **Figure 6-6E** and **Figure 6-6F**. You need to move the left heel outward so that the left knee is in line with the left foot. Remember: when you take the first backward step with the left foot, the right heel does not need to shift at all because the toes of the right foot are already pointed forward at the beginning of Posture Five.

Repeat the left backward step and the right backward step while playing Movement 2 one more time, respectively. Practice Backward Movement 2 four times and take four steps backward.

When you finish the last Backward Movement 2, the toes of your left foot are touching the ground, and your right foot is angled outward at 30-45 degrees, supporting the body weight. As you shift the body weight to the left leg, move your right heel outward so that the tip of your right foot will face forward. Now, you have returned to the starting posture, **Routine Stance**. You can move on to perform Closing Posture. See **Figure 6-7A**: Transition from Posture Five to Closing Posture.

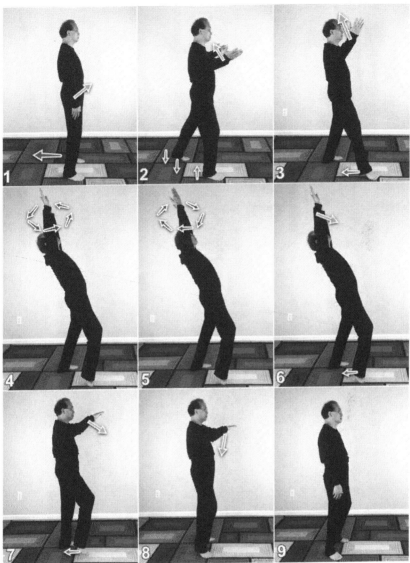

Figure 6-6B. Posture Five, the first backward step (lateral view). Walk backward and perform Backward Movement 2. (**Figure 6-6A** is placed on the following page for convenience.)

The Important Point

Bend your knees to a lesser degree or do not flex your knees at all if you feel uncomfortable or pain in Routine Stance, Transitional Stance, or Empty Stance.

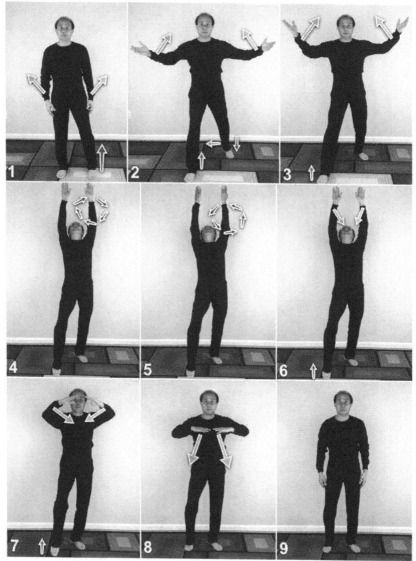

Figure 6-6A. Posture Five, the first backward step (front view). Walk backward and perform Backward Movement 2.

Key points for **Figure 6-6A** and **Figure 6-6B**.

Photo #1: At the conclusion of Posture Four, you are back in **Transitional Stance** with the right leg supporting the body and ready to step back with your left foot. **Photo #2**: Step backward with your left foot while circling your hands up to the sides (**Movement 2**). As the toes of your left foot are touching the ground, gradually shift the weight to the left leg while you continue to raise your hands. At this moment, your hands are at shoulder level. And your left heel will be naturally moved inward as the whole foot contacts the ground. **Inhale** while raising your hands.

Photo #3: Continue to circle your hands up and start to look upward. Your left foot (the rear foot) is in complete contact with the ground. Your right heel (the front foot) comes off the ground as your weight has entirely shifted to the left leg. The toes of your right foot (the front foot) are pointed forward, and the left foot (the rear foot) is angled outward at 35-45 degrees.

Photo #4: Raise your hands overhead until the arms are fully extended. At the same time, gently tilt the upper body and head backward. Keep your eyes looking upward with the palms directed forwards. Your right foot spontaneously moves backward a few inches. Now you are in **Empty Stance.** This pose looks like **Raised Arms Pose** in yoga. Hold this pose for one breath or as many breaths as you like.

Next, **exhale** and slowly rotate your arms to turn the palms backward (supinate) while keeping your arms straightened.

Photo #5: The palms have been turned backward. While staying in the pose, **inhale** and slowly rotate your arms to turn the palms forward (pronate) again.

Photo #6: The palms have been turned forward. Hereafter, slowly straighten your back and resume your upright position when you start to circle your hands down through the midline.

Photo #7: Bring your right foot back (the front foot) as you continue to lower your hands. In the meanwhile, **exhale** slowly when dropping your hands with the palms facing downward.

Photo #8: Your hands continue to descend. The right foot is positioned parallel to the left foot with the toes of the right foot touching the ground.

Photo #9: Your hands have returned to your sides. Now you are back in **Transitional Stance**: your left leg is supporting your weight while the toes of your right foot gently touch the ground to keep balance. You are ready to continue the backward step with the right foot and proceed to perform the next Movement 2. See **Figure 6-6E** and **Figure 6-6F**.

Breathing Coordination. Photos #1, **#2**, and **#3**: Inhale while raising the hands. **Photo #4**: Exhale while turning the palms backward (supinate). **Photo #5**: Inhale while turning the palms forward (pronate). **Photos #6**, **#7**, and **#8**: Exhale while lowering the hands.

There is a minor difference between the standing and walking backward postures. See **Figure 6-6C**.

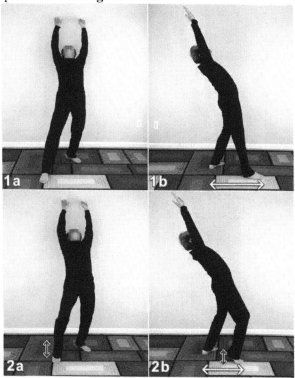

Figure 6-6C. Difference between the standing and walking backward postures. **Photos #1a** and **#1b**: In the standing backward posture, both feet maintain full contact with the ground when you are holding a pose. Please review Chapter 5 for details. **Photos #2a** and **#2b**: In the backward walking posture, the heel of the front foot (the right foot in the figure, see the vertical arrows) is off the ground, and the rear foot (the left foot) comes in full contact with the ground as you are holding a pose. In addition, the front foot (the right foot in the figure) moves backward a few inches (see the horizontal arrows).

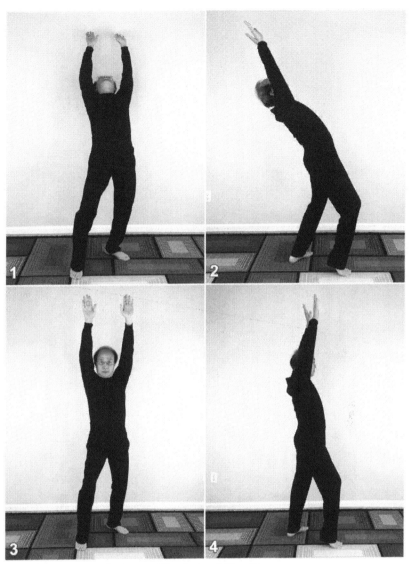

Figure 6-6D. Variations of Backward Bending.

The Important Point

Photos #1 and **#2**: Bend backward as far as you feel comfortable.

Photos #3 and **#4**: Bend backward to a lesser degree or do not bend at all if you have certain health conditions like neck/back pain, dizziness, etc.

Raise your hands to any height that is comfortable for you if you have shoulder pain or injury.

221

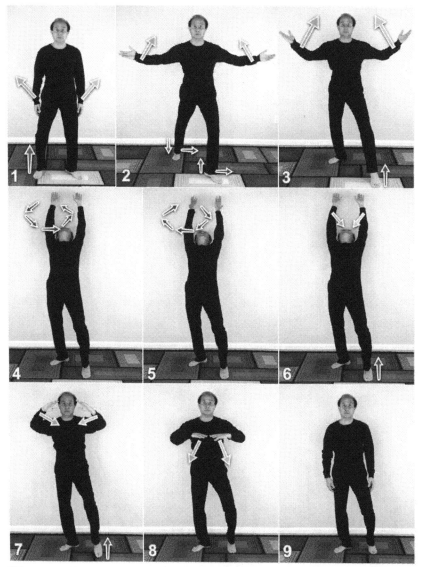

Figure 6-6E. Posture Five, the second backward step (front view).

Key points for **Figure 6-6E** and **Figure 6-6F**.

Photo #1: At the conclusion of the first Backward Movement 2, you are back in **Transitional Stance** with the left leg supporting the body and ready to step back with your right foot.

Photo #2: Step backward with your right foot while circling your hands up to the sides (**Movement 2**). **Inhale** while raising your hands.

As the toes of your right foot are touching the ground, gradually shift the weight to the right leg while you continue to raise your hands. Your hands are at shoulder level. Your left foot becomes the front foot and is angled at 30-45 degrees.

Hereafter, move the left heel outward so that the left knee is in line with the left foot. (**When you take the first backward step with your left foot, your right foot is already pointed forward. You do not need to shift the right heel.**) And your right heel will be naturally moved inward as the whole foot contacts the ground.

Photo #3: Continue to circle your hands up and start to look upward. Your right foot (the back foot) is in complete contact with the ground. After your weight has entirely shifted to the right leg, the left heel comes off the ground. At this moment, the toes of the left foot (the front foot), are pointed forward, and the right foot (the back foot) is angled outward at 35-45 degrees.

Photo #4: Raise your hands overhead until the arms are fully extended. At the same time, gently tilt the upper body and head backward. Keep your eyes looking upward with the palms directed forwards. Your left foot moves backward a few inches spontaneously. Now you are in **Empty Stance.** This pose looks like **Raised Arms Pose** in yoga. Hold this pose for one breath or as many breaths as you like.

Next, **exhale** and rotate your arms to turn the palms backward (supinate) while keeping your arms straightened.

Photo #5: The palms have been turned backward. While staying in the pose, **inhale** and slowly rotate your arms to turn the palms forward (pronate) again.

Photo #6: The palms have been turned forward. Then, **exhale** and circle your hands down through the midline. In the meanwhile, slowly straighten your back and resume your upright position.

Photo #7: Bring your front foot (the left foot) back as you continue to lower your hands with the palms facing downward.

Photo #8: Your hands continue to descend. The left foot is positioned parallel to the right foot with the toes of the left foot touching the ground.

Photo #9: Your hands have returned to your sides. Now you are back in **Transitional Stance** with your right leg supporting your weight and ready to continue the next backward step with the left foot.

Breathing Coordination. Photos #1, #2, and **#3:** Inhale while raising the hands. **Photo #4:** Exhale while turning the palms backward (supinate). **Photo #5:** Inhale while turning the palms forward (pronate). **Photos #6, #7,** and **#8:** Exhale while lowering the hands.

Carry out the same action when taking the third and fourth backward steps.

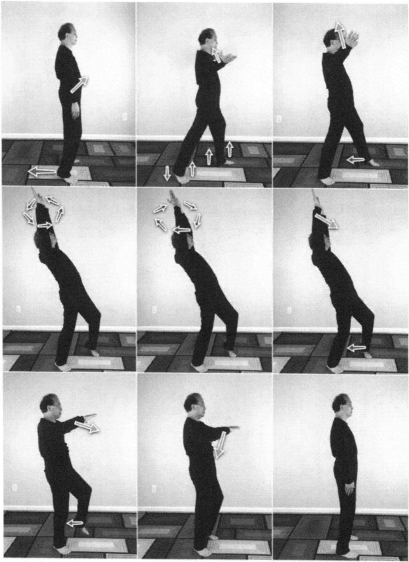

Figure 6-6F. Posture Five, the second backward step (lateral view).

Closing Posture

This posture is nothing new: Perform **Standing Downward Movement 2** four times, as described in Chapter 5. We are done!

After having finished the transition from Posture Five to Closing Posture (see **Figure 6-7A**), you are back in **Routine Stance**. Stand with your feet shoulder-width apart, your knees slightly flexed, and your hands at your sides. Now, you are ready to perform **Downward Movement 2**. See **Figure 6-7B** and **Figure 6-7C**.

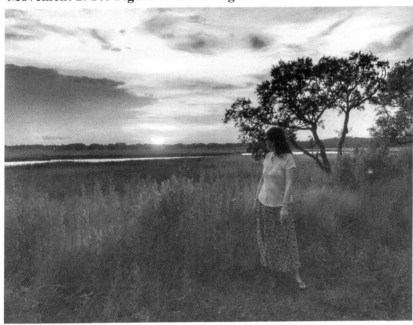

Closing Posture: Perform Downward Movement 2 **four** times while standing.

Flow Chart for Closing Posture
(Perform Movement 2 while standing.)

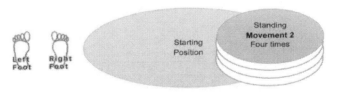

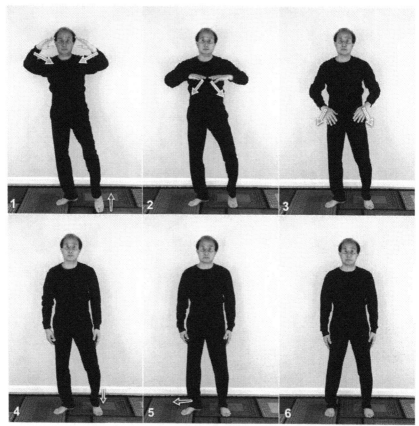

Figure 6-7A. The transition from Posture Five to Closing Posture.

Photos #1, #2, and **#3:** You are finishing the last Backward Movement 2. Please refer to **Photos #7** and **#8** in **Figure 6-6E.**

Photo #4 (Photo #9 in **Figure 6-6E):** At the conclusion of Posture Five, your right foot is angled at 30-45 degrees with the right leg supporting the body weight. The toes of the left foot are touching the ground at this moment.

Photo #5: Shift your weight to the left leg and move the right heel outward to bring your feet parallel to each other.

Photo #6: Distribute your weight evenly between both legs. Now you are back in **Routine Stance** and ready to proceed Closing Posture.

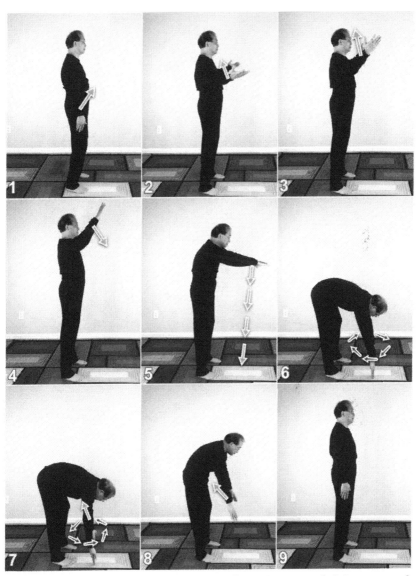

Figure 6-7C. Closing Posture: Standing Downward Movement 2 (lateral view).
(**Figure 6-7B** is placed on the following page for convenience.)

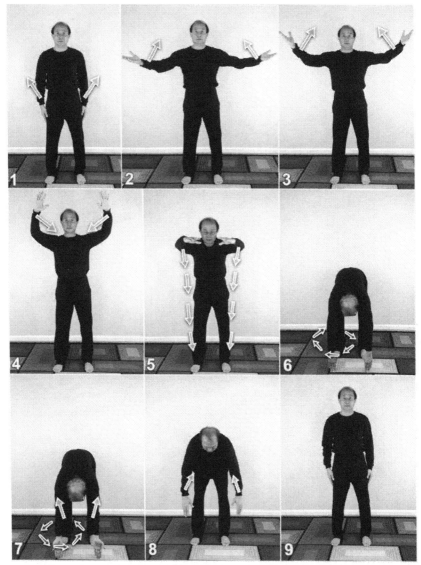

Figure 6-7B. Closing Posture: Standing Downward Movement 2 (front view).

Key points for **Figure 6-7B** and **Figure 6-7C**.

Photo #1: Start with **Routine Stance**. Stand with feet shoulder-width apart. The knees are flexed at 10-20 degrees. Your hands rest at your sides.

Photo #2: Slowly straighten your knee joints when you are raising your hands to the sides (**Movement 2**). As the arms rotate out, the palms turn progressively and face upward. **Inhale** while raising the hands. The hands are at shoulder level right now.

Photo #3: The hands continue to ascend with the palms facing upward. The palms face inward as the hands are raised above shoulder level.

Photo #4: Raise your hand overhead, or to any height you like with the palms facing forward. From now, slowly bend forward at the hips.

Photo #5: Bend forward as the hands are descending through the midline of the body. **Exhale** while lowering the hands.

Photo #6: Lower your body as far as you can with the palms facing downward and backward. Keep your knees straight if you are flexible. Otherwise, gently bend your knees and drop your hands to whatever level is comfortable for you. This pose looks like **Standing Forward Bend**. Hold the pose as long as you like.

Next, **inhale** and turn your palms forward (supinate).

Photo #7: Your palms have been turned forward.

Hereafter, **exhale** while turning your palms backward (pronate).

Photo #8: Slowly raise your body with the palms facing backward and the knees gently flexed. Continue to exhale until you resume the upright position.

Photo #9: As you resume the upright position, your hands have returned to your sides. You are back to **Routine Stance** and ready to perform the next Downward Movement 2.

Then repeat the same movement three more times.

Breathing Coordination.

Photos #1, **#2**, and **#3**: Inhale while raising the hands.

Photos #4 and #5: Exhale while lowering the hands.

Photo #6: Inhale while turning the palms forward (supinate).

Photos #7 and #8: Exhale while turning the palms backward (pronate) and returning to the upright position.

The Important Point

Do not bend at all or bend forward to a lesser degree if you have certain health conditions like back or neck pain/injury, dizziness, glaucoma, and cardiovascular diseases. See **Figure 5-3D**.

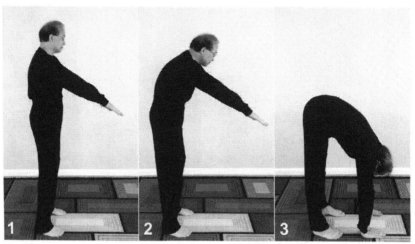

Figure 5-3D. Variations of Forward Bending.

Photo #1: Do not bend at all.

Photo #2: Bend forward to a lesser degree.

Photo #3: Touch your palms on the floor and keep your knees straight if you have good flexibility.

Yoga E Tai Chi Posture Index

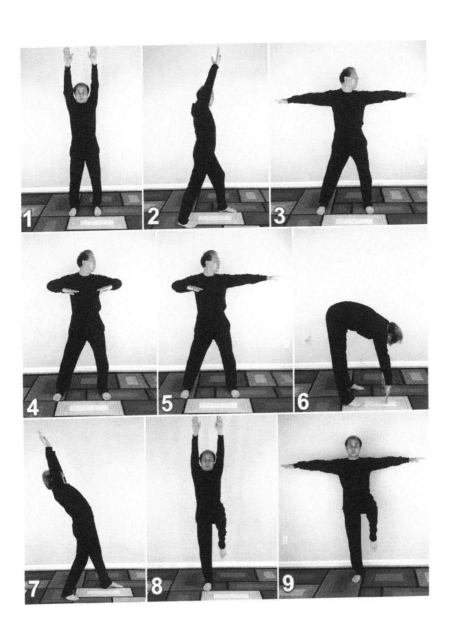

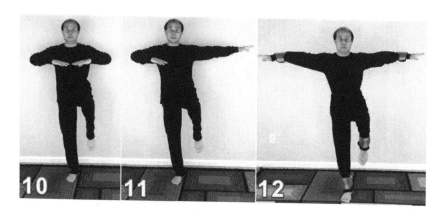

Photo #1: **Upward Movement 1** derived from **Raised Hands Pose** (Urdhva Hastasana), 130, 132, 182, 184

Photo #2: **Forward Movement 1** derived from **Warrior 1 Pose** (Virabhadrasana I), 21, 134, 136, 137, 138, 208, 210, 211, 212

Photo #3: **Sideward Movement 1** derived from **Warrior 2 Pose** (Virabhadrasana II), 68, 140, 142, 190, 193

Photo #4: **Sideward Movement 2** derived from **Mountain Pose** (Tadasana) variations, 144, 146, 196, 198

Photo #5: **Sideward Movement 3** derived from **Archer Pose**, 148, 150, 202, 204

Photo #6: **Downward Movement 2** derived from **Standing Forward Bend** (Uttanasana), 152, 154, 227, 228

Photo #7: **Backward Movement 2** derived from **Raised Arms Pose** (Hasta Uttanasana), 157, 158, 160, 161, 217, 218, 222, 224

Photo #8 Balance Movement 1a derived from **Tree Pose** (Vriksasana), 164

Photo #9: **Balance Movement 1b** derived from **Tree Pose** plus **Warrior 2 Pose**, 166

Photo #10: **Balance Movement 2** derived from a **Tree Pose** variation, 168

Photo #11: **Balance Movement 3** derived from **Tree Pose** plus **Archer Pose**, 170

Photo #12: **Postures with Weights**, 173, 174

All the postures described above can be safely and comfortably performed with wrist and ankle weights.

Epilog

授人以鱼，不如授之以渔，授人以鱼只救一时之急，授人以渔则可解一生之需。

Give a man a fish, and you feed him for a day. Teach him how to fish, and you feed him for a lifetime.

—Chinese proverb

As is the case with E Tai Chi, you can perform the Yoga E Tai Chi hand/arm movements in any direction. Moreover, your hands or arms can be overlapped (crossed over the midline of your body) and moved in large or small circles as long as you feel good. Again, there is no strict rule in Yoga E Tai Chi. You are doing the right thing if you practice it gently, comfortably, and safely. Yoga E Tai Chi is for your health only, not for fighting, competition, or spiritual purpose.

Congratulations!

After you have finished reading this book, you will obtain a valuable tool, Yoga E Tai Chi, at hand, which you can use and perfect anytime and anywhere. You can create your own Yoga E Tai Chi sequence by using the six hand movements and different ways of walking or standing. You make it, own it, and enjoy it! It will help you keep healthy, achieve peace of mind, cultivate the happiness of feeling good, and have a smile all the time. Whatever exercise you do, you should do it moderately, safely, and regularly.

Where there is a smile, there is a chance, peace, and happiness.
--Quoted from my book: ***Life and Medicine***.

Acknowledgments

I am very grateful to the following people who helped make this book a reality.

Jo, my beautiful wife, has read my book many times, comes up with many bright ideas, and continues to make caustic and funny remarks. She has taken many wonderful photos and become my first E Tai Chi student. At present, she is translating the book into Chinese. I hope that the Chinese version of the book will be published early next year. Her support and love have made my life meaningful.

Lisa Bozik, MD, my colleague, proofread two chapters of the book, provided critical comments, and corrected my English grammar errors.

William Baly, MD, my colleague, proofread one chapter and some illustrations in the book and made constructive comments.

The clinic staff support my work every day and are interested in E Tai Chi and Yoga E Tai Chi. Some of them participated in taking the gorgeous picture on the page of Yogetaichi Song. They are Trista Bonnette, Shadana Carson, Amy Coleman, Carolyn Dewitt, Kayla Easterlin, Ashley Harris, Ann Hawkins, Sarah Miller, Jami Odom, Sylvia Rush, Melanie Sheppard, Charlotte Shuler, and Amanda White.

Some of my patients put up with my yoga-tai chi teaching during office visits.

About the Author

Dr. Yongxin Li, the inventor of E Tai Chi, graduated from Guangzhou Medical College (Guangzhou Medical University) in China in the 1980s. He came to the U.S. in 1986 and received his Ph.D. degree in physiology from the University of Texas Medical Branch at Galveston in 1991. He completed his internal medicine residency at Wright State University School of Medicine in Dayton, Ohio in the 1990s. Since then, he has been practicing internal medicine in a southern state. Dr. Yongxin Li is the author of *Life and Medicine: Every Patient Teaches a Lesson*.

References

ACE Physical Therapy and Sports Medicine Institute. (2015, October 30). *Side Stepping to Treat Low Back and Lower Extremity Injuries.* Retrieved June 26, 2016, from ACE Physical Therapy and Sports Medicine Institute: http://www.ace-pt.org/2015/10/30/ace-physical-therapy-and-sports-medicine-institute-side-stepping-to-treat-low-back-and-lower-extremity-injuries/

Australian Government Department of Health. (2015). *Review of the Australian Government Rebate on Natural Therapies for Private Health Insurance.* Retrieved 11 14, 2017, from Australian Government Department of Health: http://www.health.gov.au/internet/main/publishing.nsf/Content/phi-natural-therapies

Biswas, A., Oh, P. I., Faulkner, G. E., Bajaj, R. R., Silver, M. A., Mitchell, M. S., & Alter, D. A. (2015). Sedentary Time and Its Association With Risk for Disease Incidence, Mortality, and Hospitalization in Adults: A Systematic Review and Meta-analysis. *Ann Intern Med, 162*(2), 123-132.

Broad, W. J. (2012). *The Science of Yoga The Risks and the Rewards.* Simon & Schuster.

Broad, W. J. (2012, Feburary 27). *Yoga and Sex Scandals: No Surprise Here.* Retrieved from The New York Times: http://www.nytimes.com/2012/02/28/health/nutrition/yoga-fans-sexual-flames-and-predictably-plenty-of-scandal.html

Bryant, M. S., Workman, C. D., Hou, J.-G. G., Henson, H. K., & York, M. K. (2016). Acute and Long-Term Effects of Multidirectional Treadmill Training on Gait and Balance in Parkinson Disease. *PM R, 8*(12), 1151-1158.

Cole, R. (2007, August 28). *Protect the Knees in Lotus and Related Postures.* Retrieved from Yoga Journal:

https://www.yogajournal.com/teach/protect-the-knees-in-lotus-and-related-postures

Cramer, H., Krucoff, C., & Dobos, G. (2013). Adverse Events Associated with Yoga: A Systematic Review of Published Case Reports and Case Series. *PLoS One, 8*(10), e75515.

Cramer, H., Ostermann, T., & Dobos, G. (2017, September 20). Injuries and other adverse events associated with yoga practice: A systematic review of epidemiological studies. *J Sci Med Sport, 17*(3), S1440-2440.

Cramer, H., WardL, L., Saper, R., Fishbein, D., Dobos, G., & Lauche, R. (2015). The Safety of Yoga: A Systematic Review and Meta-Analysis of Randomized Controlled Trials. *American Journal of Epidemiology, 182*(4), 281-93.

Diaz, K. M., Howard, V. J., Hutto, B., Natalie, C., Vena, J. E., Safford, M. M., . . . Hooker, S. P. (2017). Patterns of Sedentary Behavior and Mortality in U.S. Middle-Aged and Older Adults: A National Cohort Study. *Ann Intern Med.*

Dicharry, J. (2010). Kinematics and kinetics of gait: from lab to clinic. *Clin Sports Med, 29*(3), 347-64.

Feuerstein, G. (2013). *The Yoga Tradition: It's History, Literature, Philosophy and Practice* . Hohm Press.

Fishman, L. (2014). *Healing Yoga: Proven Postures to Treat Twenty Common Ailments—from Backache to Bone Loss, Shoulder Pain to Bunions, and More.* W. W. Norton & Company.

Fu (Author), Z., & Swaim (Translator), L. (2012). *Mastering Yang Style Taijiquan.* Blue Snake Books.

Gilchrist, L. (1998). Age-related changes in the ability to side-step during gait. *Clin Biomech*, 91-97.

Grant, K.-L. (2015, FEBRUARY 17). *A List of Yoga Scandals Involving Gurus, Teachers, Students, Sex and Other Inappropriate Behaviour.* Retrieved 10 31, 2017, from The Yoga Lunchbox: https://theyogalunchbox.co.nz/acompehrensive-list-of-yoga-scandals-involving-gurus-sex-and-other-inappropriate-behaviour/

Handford, M. L., & Srinivasan, M. (2014). Sideways walking: preferred is slow, slow is optimal, and optimal is expensive. *Biol Lett., 10*(1), 20131006.

Hempel, S., Taylor, S. L., R, S. M., Miake-Lye, I. M., Beroes, J. M., Shanman, R., & Shekelle, P. G. (2014). *Evidence Map of Tai Chi.* Washington (DC): Department of Veterans Affairs (US).

Herrington, S. (2017, June 7). *Yoga Teachers Need a Code of Ethics.* Retrieved October 21, 2017, from The New York Times: https://www.nytimes.com/2017/06/07/opinion/yoga-code-of-ethics-bikram-choudhury.html

Huffpost. (2017, June 21). *Narendra Modi Performs Yoga In Rain, Says The Practice Has Played A Big Role In Binding The World.* Retrieved October 21, 2017, from Huffpost: http://www.huffingtonpost.in/2017/06/21/narendra-modi-performs-yoga-in-rain-says-the-practice-has-playe_a_22494537/

Iyengar, B. K. (1995). *Light on Yoga: The Bible of Modern Yoga.* Schocken.

Johns Hopkins Medicine. (n.d.). *Vital Signs.* Retrieved 11 14, 2017, from Johns Hopkins Medicine: https://www.hopkinsmedicine.org/healthlibrary/conditions/cardiovascular_diseases/vital_signs_body_temperature_pulse_rate_respiration_rate_blood_pressure_85,P00866

Khalsa, S. B., Cohen, L., Mcall, T., & Telles, S. (2016). *Principles and Practice of Yoga in Health Care.* HANDSPRING PUBLISHING.

Kim, T.-W., & Kim, Y.-W. (2014). Treadmill Sideways Gait Training with Visual Blocking for Patients with Brain Lesions. *J Phys Ther Sci., 26* (9), 1415–1418.

Lear, S., Gasevic, D., & Hu, W. (2016). The effect of overall and types of physical activity on mortality and cardiovascular events in 17 countries: Results from the Prospective Urban Rural Epidemiologic (PURE) study. *World Congress of Cardiology & Cardiovascular Health*, (p. Abstract OC01_02). Mexico City, Mexico.

Li, Y. (2015). *Life and Medicine.* Amazon Digital Services LLC.

Liu, T., & Qiang, X. M. (2013). *Chinese Medical Qigong .* Singing Dragon.

Li 李德印, D. (2003). *太极拳规范教程 (The Textbook of Standardized Taijiquan).* 人民体育出版社.

Lowes, R. (2017, May 12). *Opioid Makers May Have to Teach Physicians About Yoga.* Retrieved from Medscape: http://www.medscape.com/viewarticle/879979

Maki, B. E., & McIlroy, W. E. (2006). Control of rapid limb movements for balance recovery: age-related changes and implications for fall prevention. *Age Ageing, 35* (Suppl), ii12-ii18.

Matsushita, T., & Oka, T. (2015). A large-scale survey of adverse events experienced in yoga classes. *Biopsychosoc Medicine, 9*(9).

McCall, T. (2007). *Yoga as Medicine: The Yogic Prescription for Health and Healing.* Bantam.

Men 门, H. (2011). *东岳太极拳 （Dongyue Taijiquan）.* 人民体育出版社.

Mourdoukoutas, P. (2012, 1 14). *The Ten Golden Rules on Living the Good Life.* Retrieved 8 20, 2016, from Forbes.com: http://www.forbes.com/sites/panosmourdoukoutas/2012/01/14/the-ten-golden-rules-on-living-the-good-life/#21ac926a5c82

Nahin, R. L., Boineau, R., Khalsa, P. S., Stussman, B. J., & Weber, W. J. (2016, September). Evidence-Based Evaluation of Complementary Health Approaches for Pain Management in the United States. *Mayo Clinic Proceedings, 91*(9), 1292–1306.

Oaklander, M. (2016, September 12). The New Science of Exercise. *TIME*, p. 54.

Penman, S., Cohen, M., Stevens, P., & Jackson, S. (2012). Yoga in Australia: Results of a national survey. *Int J Yoga, 5*(2), 92-101.

Rama, S. (1992). *Meditation and Its Practice.* Himalayan Institute Press.

Rama, S. (2002). *Samadhi: The Highest State of Wisdom.* Lotus Press.

Rama, S. (2009). *Science of Breath: A Practical Guide.* Himalayan Institute Press.

Robin, M. (2017). *A 21st-Century Yogasanalia: Celebrating the Integration of Yoga, Science, and Medicine.* Wheatmark, Inc.

Rose, J. (n.d.). *Clinical Gait Analysis.* Retrieved 8 28, 2016, from https://web.stanford.edu/class/engr110/2009/Rose-08a.pdf

Saper, R. B., Lemaster, C., Delitto, A., & al, e. (2017). Yoga, Physical Therapy, or Education for Chronic Low Back Pain: A Randomized Noninferiority Trial. *Ann Intern Med, 167*(2), 85-94.

Saraswati, S. N. (2016). *Prana and Pranayama.* Yoga Publications Trust.

Statista. (n.d.). *Number of participants in Tai Chi in the United States from 2008 to 2015 (in millions).* Retrieved September 2, 2017, from Statista: https://www.statista.com/statistics/191622/participants-in-tai-chi-in-the-us-since-2008/

Swain, T. A., & McGwin, G. (2016). Yoga-Related Injuries in the United States From 2001 to 2014. *Orthop J Sports Med, 4* (11), 2325967116671703.

The United States Department of Veterans Affairs. (n.d.). *Clinical Staff Guide to Pedometers - Move!* Retrieved 8 28, 2016, from http://www.move.va.gov/docs/Resources/ClinicalStaffGuideToPedometer2011.pdf

The University of Washington. (n.d.). *Gait I: Overview, Overall Measures, and Phases of Gait.* Retrieved 8 28, 2016, from courses.washington.edu/.:

http://courses.washington.edu/anatomy/KinesiologySylla bus/GaitPhasesKineticsKinematics.pdf

Wang, C., Schmid, C. H., Iversen, M. D., Harvey, W. F., Fielding, R. A., Driban, J. B., . . . McAli, T. (2016). Comparative Effectiveness of Tai Chi Versus Physical Therapy for Knee Osteoarthritis: A Randomized Trial. *Ann Intern Med, 165*(2), 77-86.

Wayne, P. M., & Fuerst, M. L. (2013). *The Harvard Medical School Guide to Tai Chi: 12 Weeks to a Healthy Body, Strong Heart, and Sharp Mind (Harvard Health Publications) Kindle Edition.* Shambhala Publications.

Wayne, P. M., Berkowitz, D. L., Litrownik, D. E., Buring, E, J., & Yeh, G. Y. (2014). What do we really know about the ot of tai chi?: A systemic review of adverse event reports in randomized trials. *Arch Phys Med Rehabil*, 2477-83.

Wei, M., & Groves, J. (2017). *The Harvard Medical School Guide to Yoga: 8 Weeks to Strength, Awareness, and Flexibility.* Da Capo Lifelong Books.

Yackle, K., Schwarz, L. A., Kam, K., Sorokin, J. M., .Huguenard, J. R., Feldman, J. L., . . . Krasnow, M. A. (2017). Breathing control center neurons that promote arousal in mice. *Science. 2017, 355*(6332), 1411-1415.

Yan, J., Gu, W., Sun, J., Zhang, W., Li, B., & Pan, L. (2013). Efficacy of Tai Chi on pain, stiffness and function in patients with osteoarthritis: a meta-analysis. *PLoS One, 8*(4), e61672.

Yang, J.-M. (2015). *Tai Chi Qigong: The Internal Foundation of Tai Chi Chuan.* YMAA Publication Center.

Yoga Journal. (2016, January 13). *2016 Yoga in America Study Conducted by Yoga Journal and Yoga Alliance Reveals Growth and Benefits of the Practice.* Retrieved September 2, 2017, from Yoga Journal: https://www.yogajournal.com/page/yogainamericastudy

Yuan 苑显英, X. (2014). *成都市区太极拳练习者膝关节痛现状的调查与分析 (A Study of Knee Pain in Taijiquan Practitioners in Chengdu, China).* Retrieved 9 4, 2016,

from 中国知网(cnki):
http://cdmd.cnki.com.cn/Article/CDMD-10653-1014364342.htm

Zeng, Y., Luo, T., Xie, H., Huang, M., & Cheng, A. (2014). Health benefits of qigong or tai chi for cancer patients: a systematic review and meta-analyses. *Complement Ther Med, 22*((1)), 173-86.

Zhu, D., Li, L., Qiu, P., Wang, S., Xie, Y., & Chen, X. (2011). 上海市区太极拳练习者膝关节疼痛调查分析 (A Survey on Knee Pain of Tai Chi Quan Practitioners in Shanghai Urban Area). *中国运动医学杂志 (Chin J Sports Med), 30*(9), 825-829.

Made in the USA
Columbia, SC
18 April 2021